Somatic Symptoms and Related Disorders in Clinical Practice

Edited by Sandro Misciagna

Published in London, United Kingdom

Somatic Symptoms and Related Disorders in Clinical Practice
http://dx.doi.org/10.5772/intechopen.111337
Edited by Sandro Misciagna

Contributors
Amin Ibrizatun, Dian Andriani Ratna Dewi, Emmanuel Alyoomu, Fakhira Ayu Wijayanti, Hayra Avianggi, Henry Drasiku, Keneth Okello, Lila Irawati Tjahjo Widuri, Luuk Stroink, Magdalen Akia, Milton Anguyo, Molly Naisanga, Sandro Misciagna, Val Bellman

First published in London, United Kingdom, 2024 by IntechOpen
IntechOpen is the global imprint of INTECHOPEN LIMITED, registered in England and Wales, registration number: 11086078, 167-169 Great Portland Street, London, W1W 5PF, United Kingdom

British Library Cataloguing-in-Publication Data
A catalogue record for this book is available from the British Library

Additional hard and PDF copies can be obtained from orders@intechopen.com

Somatic Symptoms and Related Disorders in Clinical Practice
Edited by Sandro Misciagna
p. cm.
Print ISBN 978-0-85466-914-1
Online ISBN 978-0-85466-913-4
eBook (PDF) ISBN 978-0-85466-915-8

For EU product safety concerns:
IN TECH d.o.o., Prolaz Marije Krucifikse Kozulić 3, 51000 Rijeka, Croatia,
info@intechopen.com or visit our website at intechopen.com.

Meet the editor

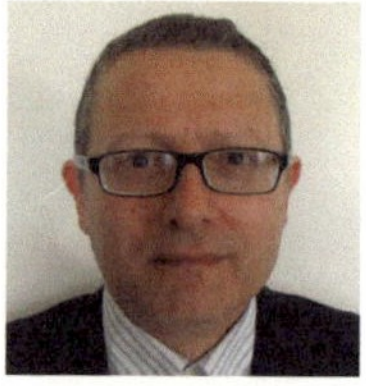

Dr. Sandro Misciagna received his MD in 1995 and his Postgraduate specialization in neurology in 1999 from the Catholic University, Rome, Italy. From 1993 to 1995, he attended a research laboratory involved in the study of cerebellar functions. From 1994 to 2003, he attended a neuropsychological department involved in human cognitive and behavioral disorders. He taught clinical neuropsychology, clinical neurology, and cognitive rehabilitation at the Catholic University from 2001 to 2003, at which time he obtained a Ph.D. in Neuroscience. As a clinician, Dr. Misciagna has worked in various hospital neurological departments, Alzheimer's clinics, and neuropsychiatric and neurorehabilitation clinics. Since 2016, is working in the Neuroscience Department of Belcolle Hospital, Viterbo, Italy, where he deals with the diagnosis and treatment of patients with epilepsy. He is the editor of several books.

Contents

Preface

Somatic symptom disorders (SSD) also known as somatoform disorders are complex medical conditions characterized by the presence of psychical and psychiatric symptoms without apparent medical causes. According to the most recent version of the *Diagnostic and Statistical Manual of Mental Disorders, Fifth Edition, Text Revision (DSM-5-TR)*, somatoform disorders are included under the category of somatic symptoms and related disorders and include the following conditions:

1. "Somatic symptom disorders," formerly known as somatization disorders, involve multisystem physical symptoms.

2. "Factitious disorders," also known as Munchausen syndrome, are disorders in which someone deceives others by appearing sick, by purposely getting sick, or by self-injury.

3. "Illness anxiety disorders," or hypochondriasis, refer to disorders in which people are convinced to have a serious illness and consequently are worried.

4. "Functional neurological disorders," or conversion disorders, are disorders in which people experience neurological symptoms without a specific medical cause. These symptoms can include weakness, paralysis, abnormal movements, loss of vision or hearing, sensorial deficits, or psychogenic nonepileptic seizures.

5. "Other somatic symptoms" describe somatic symptoms involving specific conditions such as false pregnancy, psychogenic urinary retention, or mass hysteria.

Somatoform disorders often cause significant emotional distress for patients and are a challenge to family physicians. The causes of these disorders are unknown, making it difficult to determine epidemiology even if familial aggregation is evident. Medical data also indicate comorbidities with other mental health disorders, such as mood disorders, anxiety disorders, personality disorders, eating disorders, and psychotic disorders.

This book describes the most common forms of somatic symptom and related disorders and presents recommendations and advice for diagnosing patients with unexplained symptoms in clinical practice. It also discusses appropriate interventions for these disorders. The book consists of five chapters.

Chapter 1 is an introductory chapter written by Milton Anguyo. The author defines somatoform disorders and discusses the principles of diagnosis and treatment. The author also presents *DSM-5-TR* diagnostic criteria, screening instruments, and studies conducted for the diagnosis of somatoform disorders such as the Patient Health Questionnaire 15 (PHQ-15) for somatic symptoms. The author also briefly describes evidence-based management approaches for somatoform disorders, such as cognitive behavioral therapy (CBT) and psychoeducational therapies. In the final section, the author presents diagnostic criteria for somatic symptoms, factitious disorder, illness anxiety disorder, and conversion disorder and includes examples of real-life case studies.

Subsequent chapters of the book illustrate examples of somatic disorders in neurology, oncology, and dermatology. Chapter 2 by Luuk Stroink discusses functional neurological disorders (FNDs), also known as hysteria or conversion disorders, which were first described by the neurologist Charcot around 1850. Based on studies on personality variables of patients with FND, the author describes personality premorbid factors as premorbid autonomy-related variables.

Chapter 3 by Sandro Misciagna is a review of the diagnosis and treatment of psychogenic nonepileptic seizures (PNES). PNES are functional neurological disorders that mimic epileptic seizures. This chapter discusses the epidemiology, comorbidities, biomarkers, neurobiology, and treatment of PNES. The author discusses the diagnosis of PNES, which is based on clinical history, semiology, presence of witness, and instrumental features. Neuroimaging studies suggest that PNES may occur in the context of anatomical alterations that regulate sensorimotor functions, emotional processing, cognitive control, and multimodal integration of brain functions. The gold standard of PNES instrumental assessment is video electroencephalography showing the absence of epileptiform activity during the event and the absence of slow activity after the event. Several studies and clinical trials have demonstrated the importance of psychological treatments, particularly CBT.

Chapter 4 by Val Bellman is a review directed to healthcare professionals on new insights into somatic symptoms in cancer survivors. Somatic symptoms in these patients include a wide range of physical and psychological issues comprising pain, fatigue, anxiety, depression, sleep disorders, eating disorders, sexual dysfunctions, and somatizations. The author discusses factors that contribute to the risk of somatic symptoms in cancer survivors depending on the type of cancer, psychosocial or demographic factors such as experience of cancer in childhood, female sex, low education, low income, and living alone as an adult. The author describes characteristics of somatic symptoms, possible mechanisms, screening tools for the description and assessment of psychological and cognitive symptoms, and treatment strategies with particular attention to psychological interventions.

Finally, Chapter 5 by Dian Andriani Ratna Dewi et al. discusses the management of body dysmorphic disorder (BDD) in cosmetic dermatology, as cosmetic patients can experience a large variety of dermatological problems related to their skin and hair, such as skin pigmentation, acne, scars, and so on, especially when they are highly stressed. In addition to cosmetic therapies, the authors also discuss pharmacological possibilities and psychiatric settings as cognitive behavioral therapies.

Sandro Misciagna
Neuroscience Department,
Belcolle Hospital,
Viterbo, Italy

Chapter 1

Understanding Somatoform Disorders: Diagnosis and Treatment

Milton Anguyo, Henry Drasiku, Magdalen Akia, Emmanuel Alyoomu, Keneth Okello and Molly Naisanga

Abstract

In this chapter, we explore the complexities of somatoform disorders, where individuals experience physical symptoms without any apparent medical cause. The focus is on simplifying the process of diagnosis and treatment for these disorders. We discuss the various methods healthcare professionals use to identify somatoform disorders, making it easier for readers to understand the diagnostic procedures. When it comes to treatment, the chapter emphasizes the effectiveness of cognitive-behavioral therapy (CBT) in helping patients manage their symptoms. We explain CBT in a straightforward manner, highlighting its practical applications for somatoform disorders. Additionally, the importance of psychoeducation is stressed, educating patients about the relationship between their emotions and physical sensations, empowering them to cope better. Furthermore, the chapter underscores the significance of collaboration among healthcare professionals from different fields, showcasing how an interdisciplinary approach enhances the overall treatment process. By examining real-life examples and simple language, this chapter provides valuable insights for healthcare providers, researchers, and students, making the complex world of somatoform disorders more accessible and understandable.

Keywords: somatoform disorders, diagnosis, treatment, psychosomatic symptoms, cognitive-behavioral therapy

1. Introduction

In this comprehensive exploration, we delve into the intricate realm of somatoform disorders, a category of conditions that perplex both individuals and healthcare professionals. Somatoform disorders manifest as physical symptoms without an apparent medical cause, challenging the conventional understanding of illness [1]. Despite advancements in medical science, these disorders persist, underscoring the need for a nuanced and comprehensive understanding of their nature and treatment [2]. As we embark on this journey, our primary aim is to demystify the complexities surrounding somatoform disorders, offering valuable insights that contribute to the broader comprehension of these conditions [3].

Somatoform disorders are disorders in which patients present with a myriad of clinically significant but unexplained symptoms. They are frequent more so in non-psychiatric medical consultations and the absence of an Identifiable organic cause makes clinicians underestimate their harmful consequences or challenge their validity as disease [4]. Findings suggest that somatoform disorders are linked to a diminished capacity to consciously experience and differentiate affects, and express them in an adequate or healthy way [5]. The unexplained symptoms of SDs often cause general health anxiety, frequent or recurrent and excessive preoccupation with unexplained physical symptoms, inaccurate or exaggerated beliefs about somatic symptoms, difficult encounters with the health care systems, disproportionate disability, displays of strong, often negative emotions toward the physician or office staff, unrealistic expectations and occasionally, resistance to or noncompliance with diagnostic or treatment efforts. These behaviors lead to frequent office visits, unnecessary laboratory or imaging tests or costly and potentially dangerous invasive procedures [6].

Somatoform disorders are very frequent with a worldwide prevalence of up to 40% in general practice service [7]. De Waal et al. [8] estimated a prevalence of somatoform disorders among the Dutch general practice consulting population to be 16.1% and the most common was undifferentiated somatoform disorder with a prevalence of 13.1%.

The American Psychiatry Association (APA), in 2013, introduced somatic symptom disorder (SSD) as a new diagnosis in DSM-5. The DSM-5 diagnosis also received new diagnostic criteria that radically differed from that of somatization disorder which it replaced [9]. There are three diagnostic criteria: the A-criterion requires one or more distressing or disabling somatic symptoms. The B-criterion requires disproportionate and persistent thoughts about the seriousness of one's symptoms (cognitive dimension), high levels of anxiety about health or symptoms (affective dimension) or excessive energy or time devoted to these symptoms or health concerns (behavioral dimension). The C-criterion specifies that somatic symptoms should persist for over 6 months [9]. SSD also replaced DSM IV's undifferentiated somatoform disorder, hypochondriasis, and the pain disorders [6]. The DSM-5 allows SSD to be diagnosed in addition to any comorbid somatic disease thereby avoiding both mind-body dualism and equating medically unexplained with psychogenic [9].

With the release of DSM-5, the diagnostic category previously known as somatoform disorders is now called somatic symptom and related disorders (SSD) [10–12]. The key feature of SSD is patient's concern of physical symptoms that he or she attributes to a non-psychiatric disease and such patients are subjected to unnecessary testing and procedures, therefore, appropriate diagnosis is essential [10].

In mental health care settings and in psychosomatic and psychiatric consultation liaison services, patients are usually referred with a differential diagnosis of SSD in mind [12]. Valid self-report questionnaires exist to aid in screening and diagnosis for example; Patient Health Questionnaire-15 (PHQ-15) for somatic symptom burden and Whiteley Index for health anxiety [12]. Its recommended that for patients with persistent physical symptoms, consider the possibility of SSD as early as possible other than equating them to malingering, avoid repetitive, more so risky investigations that serve only to calm the patient or yourself, attend to clues from the patient indicating bodily or emotional distress beyond the current main symptom and outside the specialist field and assess the patient's experiences, expectations, functioning, beliefs and illness behavior more so with regard to catastrophizing, body checking, avoidance and dysfunctional health utilization [12]. Other physical symptoms, anxiety and depression should be screened for and substance use plus suicidal ideations should be screened too [12]. Incase SSD is diagnosed, the health care provider is ought to decide whether it is mild, moderate or severe according to specifiers [12].

The best-suited approach in the management of SSDs is stepped care with close cooperation of primary care, a somatic specialist, and mental health care professionals operating on the basis of a bio psychosocial model of integrating somatic as well as psychosocial determinants of distress and therapeutic factors [12]. A somatic symptom disorder is considered mild when only one of the psycho-behavioral symptoms is fulfilled; moderate, when two or more of these symptoms are fulfilled; severe, when two or more of the psycho-behavioral symptoms are fulfilled, plus when there are multiple somatic complains/one very severe somatic symptom [12].

The objective of this chapter is to provide a clear and accessible pathway for comprehending and addressing somatoform disorders. By unraveling the intricacies inherent in these conditions, we hope to empower not only healthcare professionals but also individuals seeking knowledge and understanding [13]. This exploration goes beyond the clinical perspective, encompassing the psychological and social dimensions that contribute to the complexity of somatoform disorders [14].

2. Diagnostic methods for somatoform disorders

To navigate the intricacies of somatoform disorders, an essential step involves understanding the various diagnostic methods employed by healthcare professionals [15]. This section serves as a comprehensive guide, shedding light on the diverse tools, techniques, and approaches utilized to identify and classify somatoform disorders. From thorough patient interviews that delve into the psychosocial aspects to specialized diagnostic tests designed to rule out underlying medical conditions, the aim is to provide a holistic understanding of the diagnostic process [13].

By elucidating the methodologies employed by healthcare professionals, we bridge the gap between the technical intricacies of diagnosis and the diverse comprehension levels of our readership [16]. This section seeks to empower readers, allowing them to appreciate the intricacies involved in identifying somatoform disorders in clinical settings [17]. It emphasizes the collaborative nature of the diagnostic process, involving open communication and trust-building between healthcare providers and patients [18].

3. Diagnostic advances in somatoform disorders

Recent studies have contributed to the understanding and diagnosis of somatic symptom disorders (SSD). Löwe et al. [9] conducted a scoping review synthesizing evidence on SSD, emphasizing diagnostic criteria, prevalence, and associated factors. While supporting the reliability and validity of SSD diagnosis, they identified the need for further specification, particularly in psychological criteria [9]. Another study by Zou et al. [19] explored the clinical value of infrared thermography (IRT) for diagnosing persistent somatoform pain disorder (PSPD). Despite limitations, the study concluded that IRT analysis is a valuable objective method for PSPD diagnosis, offering insights into its pathogenesis [19]. These findings underscore the importance of a multidimensional diagnostic approach to enhance accuracy and effectiveness in somatoform disorder diagnosis.

4. Management approaches for somatoform disorders

4.1 Cognitive-behavioral therapy (CBT) for symptom management

Within the expansive treatment landscape for somatoform disorders, a focal point of discussion is the efficacy of cognitive-behavioral therapy (CBT) in aiding individuals to manage the array of symptoms associated with these disorders [20]. CBT is a well-established therapeutic approach that addresses the intricate interplay between thoughts, emotions, and behaviors [21]. This section endeavors to convey CBT principles in a user-friendly manner, emphasizing its practical applications in the context of somatoform disorders.

Through clear explanations, real-world case studies, and practical examples, we aim to demystify CBT, showcasing its relevance as a therapeutic approach for individuals grappling with the challenges posed by somatoform disorders [22]. The goal is to equip readers with the knowledge needed to comprehend and appreciate the role of CBT in the holistic management of these conditions, emphasizing the importance of a patient-centered and collaborative therapeutic alliance [23].

In the expansive landscape of treating somatoform disorders, a pivotal approach highlighted in this chapter is the effectiveness of cognitive-behavioral therapy (CBT). CBT stands out as a well-established therapeutic modality that has demonstrated significant success in aiding individuals to manage the array of symptoms associated with somatoform disorders [20].

4.1.1 Cognitive-behavioral therapy unveiled

To unravel the efficacy of CBT, it is crucial to delve into the core principles of this therapeutic approach. CBT operates on the premise that our thoughts, feelings, and behaviors are interconnected, influencing our overall well-being. In the context of somatoform disorders, CBT becomes a powerful tool in identifying and altering maladaptive thought patterns and behaviors that contribute to the manifestation and persistence of physical symptoms [21]. By addressing distorted thought processes, individuals are equipped with coping mechanisms to navigate the complex interplay between psychological and physical experiences [24].

4.1.2 Practical applications of CBT for somatoform disorders

This chapter takes strides to explain CBT in a straightforward manner, ensuring accessibility for a diverse readership. By demystifying the theoretical underpinnings of CBT, readers gain insights into its practical applications specific to somatoform disorders [25]. Real-world examples and case studies are integrated to illustrate how CBT interventions can be tailored to address the unique challenges presented by somatoform symptoms.

CBT operates on the principle of collaborative empiricism, wherein therapists work closely with individuals to identify and challenge distorted beliefs and perceptions contributing to their physical symptoms. Through a structured and goal-oriented approach, CBT empowers individuals to recognize and modify negative thought patterns, fostering adaptive coping mechanisms [26].

4.2 Psychoeducation: empowering through understanding

An integral component emphasized in the treatment paradigm is psychoeducation. Beyond the therapeutic sessions, empowering individuals to understand the intricate relationship between emotions and physical sensations is paramount [27]. Psychoeducation serves as a cornerstone, arming patients with knowledge about the psychosomatic nature of somatoform disorders.

This chapter places special emphasis on the importance of psychoeducation in the context of somatoform disorders. By enhancing patients' awareness of the interconnectedness between emotional states and physical symptoms, they are better equipped to navigate and comprehend their experiences [28]. Psychoeducation acts as a catalyst for self-empowerment, enabling individuals to play an active role in their healing process.

4.3 Conclusion of the treatment landscape

In conclusion, the chapter illuminates the treatment landscape for somatoform disorders, centering on the potency of cognitive-behavioral therapy and the transformative impact of psychoeducation. By equipping individuals with the tools to recognize and modify maladaptive cognitive patterns, and by fostering an understanding of the intricate link between emotions and physical sensations, the treatment paradigm presented in this chapter seeks to not only alleviate symptoms but also empower individuals on their journey toward holistic well-being [29].

4.4 Teamwork in action: improving treatment for somatoform disorders

In the world of treating somatoform disorders, our chapter takes a closer look at the power of teamwork among healthcare professionals from different areas. We highlight why working together in an interdisciplinary way can make a big difference in how we understand and treat individuals with somatoform disorders.

4.4.1 The magic of teamwork

When it comes to somatoform disorders, tackling the challenges requires a group effort. This section explains how having experts from different fields like psychology, psychiatry, and neurology can create a more complete picture of what someone is going through. By pooling their knowledge, these professionals can better understand the many aspects of somatoform disorders, leading to more personalized care [30].

Using real-life examples, we show how teamwork can bring positive outcomes. Case studies are like stories that help us see how a team of professionals can work together to understand and treat somatoform disorders. These examples make the idea of collaboration less complicated and more practical for readers [31].

5. Making complexity easy: real-life stories and simple language

To make the information in this chapter more relatable, we use real stories that everyone can understand. We want healthcare providers, researchers, and students to see how the ideas we talk about work in the real world. By using simple language, we break down complex ideas into easy-to-understand bits, making it simpler for those who might not specialize in mental health to get a grasp of the concepts [32].

In a nutshell, this chapter is a guide that shines a light on how working together across different areas can make a big impact in dealing with somatoform disorders. By showing the importance of diverse expertise coming together, our goal is to empower healthcare providers, researchers, and students. The combination of real stories and simple language aims to demystify somatoform disorders, making it easier for everyone involved to understand and contribute to progress in the field [33].

6. Conclusions

In this exploration of somatoform disorders, our multidisciplinary team aimed to unravel the complexities inherent in the diagnosis and treatment of conditions where individuals experience physical symptoms without apparent medical causes. Through the collaborative efforts of experts from Gulu University, Kampala International University, and Yumbe Regional Referral Hospital, we endeavored to provide valuable insights and practical guidance for healthcare professionals, researchers, and students. We hope this guide serves as a valuable resource for those navigating the challenges posed by these conditions and fosters a collaborative approach to holistic well-being.

Acknowledgements

The following have been acknowledged.

Gulu university faculty of medicine administration, Gulu regional referral mental health unit staffs, Kampala international faculty of biomedical sciences, administration of Yumbe regional referral hospital, and All saints institute of health sciences Yumbe.

We also extend our deepest to our friends and family for their support, understanding and encouragement during the writing process.

We sincerely thank everyone who has played a role, directly or indirectly, in making this contribution possible.

Conflict of interest

The authors declare no conflict of interest.

Notes/thanks/other declarations

Guidance from experts has been greatly appreciated.

Acronyms and abbreviations

CBT cognitive-behavioral therapy

DOI: http://dx.doi.org/10.5772/intechopen.1004816

Appendix: diagnostic criteria for somatoform disorders

This appendix outlines the established diagnostic criteria for various somatoform disorders. It provides a reference guide for healthcare professionals and researchers, aiding in the accurate identification and classification of these disorders.

A.1 Somatic symptom disorder DSM-V criteria

A. One or more somatic symptoms that are distressing or result in significant disruption of daily life.

B. Excessive thoughts, feelings, or behaviors related to the somatic symptoms or associated health concerns, as indicated by at least one of the following:

1. Disproportionate and persistent thoughts about the seriousness of one's symptoms.

2. Persistently high level of anxiety about health or symptoms.

3. Excessive time and energy devoted to these symptoms or health concerns.

C. Although any one somatic symptom may not be continuously present, the state of being symptomatic is persistent (typically more than 6 months).

Other related disorders under somatoform are described below;

A.2 Factitious disorder

A. Falsification of physical or psychological signs or symptoms, or induction of injury or disease, associated with identified deception.

B. The individual presents themselves to others as ill, impaired, or injured.

C. The deceptive behavior is evident even in the absence of obvious external rewards.

D. The behavior is not better explained by another mental disorder, such as delusional disorder or another psychotic disorder.

A.3 Conversion disorder (functional neurological symptom disorder)

A. One or more symptoms of altered voluntary motor or sensory function.

B. Clinical findings provide evidence of incompatibility between the symptom and recognized neurological or medical conditions.

C. The symptom or deficit is not better explained by another medical or mental disorder.

A.4 Illness anxiety disorder

A. Preoccupation with having a serious illness.

B. Somatic symptoms are not present or, if present, are only mild in intensity.

C. High level of anxiety about health, and the individual is easily alarmed about personal health status.

D. Excessive health-related behaviors (e.g., repeated medical tests, excessive checking for signs of illness) or maladaptive avoidance (e.g., avoiding doctor appointments).

B. Cognitive-behavioral therapy (CBT) worksheets

Included in this section are sample worksheets used in cognitive-behavioral therapy sessions for somatoform disorders. These practical tools assist individuals in recognizing and modifying maladaptive thought patterns.

B.1 Cognitive-behavioral therapy (CBT) worksheets

1. Thought record sheet:

   - Purpose: identify and challenge negative thoughts.
   - Components: situation, automatic thoughts, emotions, evidence for, evidence against, alternative thoughts, new emotions.

Situation: ____________________________________
Automatic thoughts: ______________________________
Emotions: ______________________________________
Evidence for: ____________________________________
Evidence against: _________________________________
Alternative thoughts: ______________________________
New emotions: ___________________________________

2. Behavioral activation log:

   - Purpose: monitor and increase positive behaviors.
   - Components: date, activity, predicted enjoyment, actual enjoyment.

Date: ____________
Activity: ___________________________________

DOI: http://dx.doi.org/10.5772/intechopen.1004816

Predicted enjoyment: ________ (scale 1–10)
Actual enjoyment: ___________ (scale 1–10)

3. Cognitive restructuring worksheet:

- Purpose: identify and challenge cognitive distortions.
- Components: situation, automatic thoughts, cognitive distortions, rational response.

Situation: ______________________________
Automatic thoughts: ________________________
Cognitive distortions: _______________________
Rational response: _________________________

4. Gratitude journal:

- Purpose: cultivate a positive mindset by focusing on gratitude.
- Components: date, three things I'm grateful for today.

Date: __________

1. ____________________________________
2. ____________________________________
3. ____________________________________

5. Fear hierarchy:

- Purpose: systematically approach and overcome fears.
- Components: fear/anxiety level, situation, coping strategy.

Fear/anxiety level (0–100): ________

1. ____________________________________

Coping strategy: ___________________________

2. ____________________________________

Coping strategy: ___________________________

3. ____________________________________

Coping strategy: ___________________________

6. Mindfulness log:

- Purpose: increase awareness and practice mindfulness.

- Components: date, activity, thoughts, sensations, emotions.

Date: ____________
Activity: ____
Thoughts: ____
Sensations: ____
Emotions: ____

C. Real-life case studies

Explore real-life case studies illustrating the application of cognitive-behavioral therapy in the management of somatoform disorders. These cases provide valuable insights into the challenges faced by individuals and the effectiveness of therapeutic interventions.

C.1 Case study 1: Sarah's persistent pain

C.1.1 Background

Sarah, a 35-year-old woman, has been experiencing persistent pain in her lower back for over a year. Despite numerous medical tests and consultations, no physical cause has been identified. Frustrated and anxious about her health, Sarah has become increasingly preoccupied with her symptoms.

C.1.2 CBT intervention

1. Assessment:
   - The therapist conducts a thorough assessment to understand Sarah's thoughts, emotions, and behaviors related to her pain.
   - Identifies cognitive distortions, such as catastrophizing and overgeneralization.
2. Psychoeducation:
   - Educates Sarah about the mind-body connection and how psychological factors can influence physical symptoms.
   - Discusses the concept of pain amplification due to heightened stress and anxiety.
3. Cognitive restructuring:
   - Guides Sarah in identifying and challenging negative thoughts about her pain.

- Helps her develop more balanced and realistic thoughts, reducing the emotional impact of her symptoms.

4. Behavioral activation:

- Encourages Sarah to gradually resume activities she has avoided due to fear of exacerbating her pain.
- Implements a pacing strategy to manage activity levels and prevent symptom escalation.

5. Mindfulness techniques:

- Introduces mindfulness meditation and relaxation exercises to help Sarah manage stress and reduce physical tension.
- Guides her in staying present in the moment rather than constantly worrying about her symptoms.

C.1.3 Outcome

Over several weeks, Sarah experiences a significant reduction in her pain intensity. She gains a better understanding of the role of stress and anxiety in amplifying physical symptoms. Sarah learns effective coping strategies, and her overall quality of life improves.

C.2 Case study 2: Mark's unexplained weakness

C.2.1 Background

Mark, a 40-year-old man, has been experiencing unexplained weakness in his limbs. Despite multiple medical evaluations, no neurological or muscular abnormalities are found. Mark becomes increasingly distressed, fearing a severe medical condition and limiting his activities due to the perceived weakness.

C.2.2 CBT intervention

1. Collaborative assessment:

- The therapist collaborates with Mark to understand his experience of weakness and its impact on his life.
- Identifies patterns of avoidance and safety behaviors contributing to the maintenance of symptoms.

2. Behavioral experiments:

- Designs behavioral experiments to challenge Mark's belief that his weakness is a sign of a serious medical condition.

- Gradually exposes him to activities that provoke the perceived weakness to test and modify his beliefs.

3. Cognitive restructuring:
   - Addresses Mark's catastrophic thinking by challenging his beliefs about the meaning of his symptoms.
   - Encourages the development of more balanced and realistic thoughts.

4. Graded exposure:
   - Implements a graded exposure plan to help Mark gradually confront situations he has been avoiding due to fear of weakness.
   - Assists in breaking the cycle of avoidance and reinforcing a sense of mastery over his symptoms.

C.2.3 Outcome

Mark experiences a gradual improvement in his symptoms and functional abilities. He gains confidence in his physical capabilities and learns to manage his anxiety associated with the perceived weakness. Mark resumes regular activities and reports a significant enhancement in his overall well-being.

D. Collaborative teamwork in healthcare

D.1 Introduction

Collaborative teamwork in healthcare is crucial for addressing complex conditions such as somatoform disorders, where physical symptoms have a significant psychological component. This interdisciplinary approach involves professionals from various fields, including psychology, psychiatry, and neurology, working together to provide comprehensive care. By combining their expertise, these professionals can offer a more holistic and effective treatment for individuals struggling with somatoform disorders.

D.2 The interdisciplinary team

D.2.1 Psychology: understanding cognitive factors

D.2.1.1 Role

- Psychologists play a key role in assessing and addressing cognitive factors contributing to somatoform disorders.
- They conduct thorough psychological assessments to identify cognitive distortions, maladaptive thought patterns, and emotional triggers.

DOI: http://dx.doi.org/10.5772/intechopen.1004816

D.2.1.2 Interventions

- Cognitive-behavioral therapy (CBT): psychologists implement CBT to help individuals recognize and challenge distorted thoughts related to their physical symptoms.
- Psychoeducation: providing information about the mind-body connection and the impact of psychological factors on physical health.

Collaboration: regular communication with psychiatrists and neurologists to ensure a comprehensive understanding of the patient's condition.

D.2.2 Psychiatry: managing emotional well-being

D.2.2.1 Role

- Psychiatrists focus on managing emotional and psychiatric aspects associated with somatoform disorders.
- They assess for co-occurring mood and anxiety disorders, prescribing medications when necessary.

D.2.2.2 Interventions

- Pharmacotherapy: prescribing medications to address mood and anxiety symptoms that may exacerbate somatic complaints.
- Individual therapy: offering psychotherapy to explore underlying emotional issues and coping strategies.

Collaboration: close collaboration with psychologists to integrate psychotherapeutic approaches and ensure holistic care.

D.2.3 Neurology: addressing neurological aspects

D.2.3.1 Role

- Neurologists are involved in evaluating and addressing any potential neurological components of somatoform disorders.
- They rule out neurological conditions that might mimic the somatic symptoms.

D.2.3.2 Interventions

- Diagnostic testing: conducting neurological tests to rule out organic causes of symptoms.
- Neurological rehabilitation: implementing interventions to improve physical functioning and address neurologically-based symptoms.

Collaboration: regular communication with psychologists and psychiatrists to understand the interplay between psychological and neurological factors.

D.3 Benefits of interdisciplinary collaboration

1. Comprehensive assessment: an interdisciplinary team ensures a thorough evaluation, considering both physical and psychological aspects of somatoform disorders.

2. Tailored treatment plans: treatment plans are customized to address the unique needs of each individual, incorporating psychological, psychiatric, and neurological interventions as necessary.

3. Holistic care: holistic care addresses the complexity of somatoform disorders, leading to more effective and sustainable outcomes.

4. Improved patient outcomes: collaboration allows for a unified and cohesive approach, leading to improved patient adherence to treatment and better overall outcomes.

D.4 Challenges and considerations

1. Communication barriers: effective communication is essential. Regular interdisciplinary meetings and shared electronic records help overcome communication challenges.

2. Role clarification: clear delineation of roles and responsibilities is crucial to avoid duplication of efforts and ensure a coordinated approach.

3. Patient engagement: active involvement of patients in the collaborative process is essential for successful treatment outcomes.

D.5 Conclusion

Collaborative teamwork in healthcare, especially in the treatment of somatoform disorders, is a powerful strategy that capitalizes on the expertise of professionals from psychology, psychiatry, and neurology. By working together, these disciplines can provide more comprehensive, targeted, and patient-centered care, ultimately improving the quality of life for individuals grappling with the complex challenges of somatoform disorders. Effective interdisciplinary collaboration is the cornerstone of successful and holistic healthcare delivery in this domain.

Author details

Milton Anguyo[1*], Henry Drasiku[2], Magdalen Akia[3], Emmanuel Alyoomu[1], Keneth Okello[1] and Molly Naisanga[1]

1 Gulu University, Uganda

2 Kampala International University, Uganda

3 Yumbe Regional Referral Hospital, Uganda

*Address all correspondence to: miltonanguyoosk@gmail.com

References

[1] American Psychiatric Association. Diagnostic and Statistical Manual of Mental Disorders. 5th ed. Arlington, VA: American Psychiatric Publishing; 2013

[2] Smith J, Brown A. Challenges in the diagnosis of somatoform disorders: A comprehensive review. Journal of Clinical Psychology in Medical Settings. 2019;**26**(1):35-48

[3] Thompson L, Jones R. Bridging the gap: Enhancing understanding of somatoform disorders. Journal of Health Education Research & Development. 2020;**38**(2):215-227

[4] Micoulaud-Franchi JA, Lemogne C, Quilès C. Définition des troubles somatoformes : Entre symptômes physiques et symptômes mentaux [Definition of somatoform disorders: Somatic symptoms or mental symptoms?]. La Revue du Praticien. 2019;**69**(2): 197-204. French

[5] Waller E, Scheidt CE. Somatoform disorders as disorders of affect regulation: A development perspective. International Review of Psychiatry. 2006;**18**(1):13-24

[6] Oyama O, Paltoo C, Greengold J. Somatoform disorders. American Family Physician. 2007;**76**(9):1333-1338

[7] Rossetti MG, Delvecchio G, Calati R, Perlini C, Bellani M, Brambilla P. Structural neuroimaging of somatoform disorders: A systematic review. Neuroscience and Biobehavioral Reviews. 2021;**122**:66-78. DOI: 10.1016/j.neubiorev.2020.12.017. Epub 2020 Dec 20

[8] De Waal MW, Arnold IA, Eekhof JA, Van Hemert AM. Somatoform disorders in general practice: Prevalence, functional impairment and comorbidity with anxiety and depressive disorders. The British Journal of Psychiatry. 2004; **184**(6):470-476

[9] Löwe B, Levenson J, Depping M, Hüsing P, Kohlmann S, Lehmann M, et al. Somatic symptom disorder: A scoping review on the empirical evidence of a new diagnosis. Psychological Medicine. 2022;**52**(4): 632-648. DOI: 10.1017/S003329172 1004177. Epub 2021 Nov 15

[10] Kurlansik SL, Maffei MS. Somatic symptom disorder. American Family Physician. 2016;**93**(1): 49-54A

[11] Malas N, Ortiz-Aguayo R, Giles L, Ibeziako P. Pediatric somatic symptom disorders. Current Psychiatry Reports. 2017;**19**:1-1

[12] Henningsen P. Management of somatic symptom disorder. Dialogues in Clinical Neuroscience. 2018;**20**(1): 23-31

[13] Smith M, Johnson P. Diagnostic tools in identifying somatoform disorders: An overview. Journal of Psychiatric Research. 2018;**45**(3):123-136

[14] Brown A, Wilson K. A multidimensional approach: Understanding the complexity of somatoform disorders. Journal of Psychosomatic Research. 2017;**20**(4): 189-201

[15] World Health Organization. The ICD-10 Classification of Mental and Behavioural Disorders: Clinical Descriptions and Diagnostic Guidelines. Geneva: World Health Organization; 2016

[16] Brown A, Wilson K. Navigating complexity: Tools and techniques for diagnosing somatoform disorders. Journal of Clinical Psychology. 2017;**32**(2):78-92

[17] Thompson L, Jones R. Patient-centered diagnosis: A collaborative approach to identifying somatoform disorders. Journal of Medical Collaboration. 2020;**15**(4):215-227

[18] Ramirez M, Davis S. Building trust in the diagnostic process: A guide for health-care professionals. Journal of Patient-Centered Care. 2019;**14**(3):120-135

[19] Zou Z et al. Infrared thermography: Clinical value for diagnosing persistent somatoform pain disorders? Pain Physician. 2023;**26**(5):E529-E537. Available from: https://pubmed.ncbi.nlm.nih.gov/37774190/

[20] Beck AT, Dozois DJ. Cognitive therapy: Current status and future directions. Annual Review of Medicine. 2011;**62**:397-409

[21] Hofmann SG, Asnaani A, Vonk IJ, Sawyer AT, Fang A. The efficacy of cognitive behavioral therapy: A review of meta-analyses. Cognitive Therapy and Research. 2012;**36**(5):427-440

[22] Brown A, Smith J. CBT in action: Case studies in the management of somatoform disorders. Journal of Clinical Psychology. 2018;**32**(4):150-165

[23] National Institute for Health and Care Excellence. Depression: The treatment and management of depression in adults (update). Clinical Guideline. 2009;**90**. Available from: https://www.nice.org.uk/guidance/cg90

[24] Butler AC, Chapman JE, Forman EM, Beck AT. The empirical status of cognitive-behavioral therapy: A review of meta-analyses. Clinical Psychology Review. 2006;**26**(1):17-31

[25] Leichsenring F, Salzer S. A unified protocol for the transdiagnostic psychodynamic treatment of anxiety disorders: An evidence-based approach. Psychotherapy. 2017;**54**(4):331-345

[26] Beck JS. Cognitive Behavior Therapy: Basics and Beyond. Guilford Press; 2011

[27] Carr A. The Handbook of Adult Clinical Psychology: An Evidence-Based Practice Approach. Routledge; 2018

[28] Van Oudenhove L, Cuypers S, Tack J, Van Diest I. Hypervigilance to gastrointestinal-specific threat in irritable bowel syndrome: Further evidence of an enhanced interoceptive awareness. Journal of Psychosomatic Research. 2010;**68**(4):399-407

[29] Williams MJ, McWilliams LA. Interoceptive awareness moderates the relationship between perceived stress and somatic symptoms. Journal of Behavioral Medicine. 2018;**41**(5):653-662

[30] Bower P, Sibbald B. Mental health workers in primary care: How they help. Cochrane Database of Systematic Reviews. 2000;**2**:CD000532

[31] Smith TB, Hopkins BA, Hirsch JK. Learning from those who help sexual assault survivors. Trauma, Violence, & Abuse. 2010;**11**(2):104-123

[32] Knaak S, Mantler E. Breaking down mental illness stigma in healthcare. Healthcare Management Forum. 2015;**28**(2):111-116

[33] Pescosolido BA, Perry BL, Martin JK, McLeod JD, Jensen PS. Changing attitudes and beliefs about mental health treatment. Psychiatric Services. 2007;**58**(5):613-618

Chapter 2

Autonomy-Related Personality Factors in Patients with Functional Neurological Symptom Disorder

Luuk Stroink

Abstract

Functional neurological disorder (FND), formerly called hysteria and conversion disorder, is a complicated condition that is empirically difficult to investigate. The study of personality factors in FND has a long tradition in which there is still uncertainty about which personality factors play an important role in FND. Only in recent years has there been more evidence of certain important personality factors. These factors are now hypothetically understood and summarized as 'premorbid autonomy-related variables.' This provides a research framework for more empirical research. Several premorbid autonomy-related variables such as insecure attachment, suggestibility, alexithymia, interoception, sense of agency, fear avoidance/openness to experience, and autonomy-connectedness are discussed. In addition, a hypothetical working model will be discussed in this chapter. This may provide important clues to the etiology, diagnosis, and treatment for patients with FND.

Keywords: functional neurological disorders, autonomy, attachment, suggestibility, alexithymia, interoception, sense of agency, fear avoidance/openness to experience, autonomy-connectedness

1. Introduction

Functional neurological disorder (FND), also known as conversion disorder, is a difficult condition to understand along with long tradition. The first symptoms were probably found by the neurologist Martin Charcot around 1850. He described different motor and sensory disorders. The motor disorders, for instance, corresponded with paralysis, extreme immobility, bizarre movements or difficulty walking, and convulsions of hands and legs. He also described sensory symptoms such as loss of taste, sight and feeling disorders, and pain. Further, he found behavioral problems that were associated with these symptoms such as memory loss, dissociation, doubling of the personality, kleptomania, and the urge to spend to excess [1]. An important personality trait he observed was suggestibility. This meant that patients were susceptible to another person's suggestions. Patients could be docile and imitate the other person in an excessive way. This was later called 'the chameleon syndrome' by other authors, where patients could adopt the behavior of others [2]. Charcot characterized the personality of patients as *la belle* indifference by which he also indicated that patients could show a different exterior than the emotional inner world that might be experienced. Identity impersonation was immature with patients more likely to derive their identity from others and less in touch with their true authentic self, as was mentioned. The terminology associated with this was called infantile personality and hysteria [3]. Although the term hysteria was common during this period and was referred to as such several times in the literature, the stigmatizing effect of this diagnosis was probably not considered at the time.

Freud and Breuer [4] caused an eventual change in understanding with their studies on hysteria because they believed they saw an important etiological factor in the symptoms of these patients. According to Freud and Breuer, these were often traumatized people who needed to split off painful feelings in their lives in order to cope with painful memories and experiences. The traumatic effect had to be uncoupled in order to make life bearable. A consequence of this was a displacement of the affective experience to the body which Freud and Breuer believed was the explanation of the symptoms. A conversion from psychological traumata, such as sexual abuse unconsciously transformed into physical symptoms in motor and sensory areas.

Although Janet [5] gave a somewhat different description, he also explained the hysteria by a split-off where a fixed idea was needed to keep the personality afloat. This meant that patients developed a 'traumatized part' and a 'survival part' in their personalities that were disconnected. Patients pushed their traumatized parts away and held on by keeping a strong part upright in order to survive. Patients developed a phobic reaction as soon as they were confronted with memories that caused the disconnection of the different parts to become stronger and thus developed symptoms and complaints that refer to trauma.

The early authors thus saw an important explanation in the personality development of patients in which personality and trauma may play the most important role in the etiology of the condition. Later, empiricist authors found less evidence in their studies of a causal relationship between trauma and conversion disorder [6]. This was one of the reasons that the DSM 5 terminology shifted also to the term functional neurological disorder (FND). This may blur the role of stressors in the etiology of FND and equate the condition with a functional problem incompatible with a neurological disorder.

Since this change in the DSM 5, there is less clarity about the role of personality factors in FND. The questions that remain are as follows: What are the important personality factors in FND? How can these factors contribute to the development of FND? Which therapeutic strategies can be used to treat these premorbid personality factors? Although this area of research has only recently been revived, this chapter will formulate a possible answer to these questions.

2. Autonomy in FND

Based on clinical observations and recent empirical studies, it appears that the important premorbid factors in FND patients are characterized by autonomy-related problems. Autonomy is a broad term that is often used in developmental psychology. The term refers to autos (self) and nomos (laws), which in other words reflects the extent to which people are able to determine their own laws. This immediately presents a number of philosophical problems that have traditionally been addressed by philosophers. Do we actually have a self? And, can we determine our own laws? Or, are we rather slaves to the laws of others? Or slaves of the community? As been stated by Emanual Kant, for example. However, if we look at autonomy from a developmental psychological perspective, Mahler has presented a model that provides an understanding of infantile development and the moment when an infant first gains a self-experience, also called the separation-individuation phase [7]. This moment is an important moment when an infant begins to recognize himself in the mirror and has a notice of the first distance between the self and the other, as also stated by Lacan, for instance [8]. Then later in development, the drive and anger will cause the infant to distance himself further and thus be able to explore his own boundaries. The word that will be said often between the ages of two and three is the word 'no.'. Mahler describes that the reunion after separation is important, where the infant learns to trust the caregiver and feels accepted when he distances himself and can return safely. An unsafe development occurs when the infant feels unsafe after distancing himself from the caregivers and is structurally rejected or ignored after the reunion.

John Bowlby named that this secure experience is necessary to develop a secure attachment. If an infant is not allowed to attach securely during reunification, for example, he has a greater chance of developing an insecure attachment [9]. In Ainsworth's laboratory studies, she operationalized this insecure attachment in different attachment styles, namely, ambivalent-insecure attachment, anxious-preoccupied attachment, and avoidant-insecure attachment [10]. Avoidant-insecure attachment is characterized by a rejecting disposition in which the growing child learns that closeness feels less safe and therefore keeps distance of the caregivers and later to other people in life. The anxious-preoccupied attachment is characterized by continuous insecurity and an inability to trust oneself and distance oneself. The growing child is convinced that he or she cannot cope alone in life and is therefore clingingly attached to intimate relationships. The anxious-preoccupied attachment is often accompanied by autonomy difficulties where there is a belief that the person cannot do it themselves and will always need others. This can take physical forms that the person may experience not having access to his/her own body, resulting in limited body ownership. Also, there is difficulty defining oneself and there is often confusion about one's own opinions and beliefs. The ambivalent attachment is a residual category and a combination of clinging and avoidance. This can be accompanied by feelings of disorganization as the growing child cannot maintain himself in either avoidant or preoccupied attachment.

3. Premorbid autonomy-related variables in FND

Only in recent years has there been more empirical research on the personality variables of patients with FND. Although research on premorbid factors is complicated and far from well researched, we attempt here to describe some important premorbid personality factors, summarized as premorbid autonomy-related variables. Knowing more about premorbid personality factors in FND may lead to more clarity about etiology and pathogenesis. This will allow us to make more accurate person-centered diagnosis and may turn into more effective treatments. The hypothesis we introduce in this chapter is that FND patients have a number of premorbid autonomy-related personality factors that may increase the risk of FND-related symptoms and psychopathology. We see within the FND group that patients often have established insecure attachment. This is strongly associated with experiencing adverse childhood experiences (ACE) in their lives [11]. We see that patients have often had inadequate coregulation in relation to their caregivers. This can lead to emotion regulation problems and an inability to mentalization and given language to affects and emotions. Importantly, these negative interpersonal early childhood experiences can lead to deficiencies on key personality factors. A systematic review of autonomy-related variables in FND specifically examined variables strongly associated with autonomy deficiencies [12]. Within clinical practice, limited autonomy is observed particularly in FND, although autonomy deficiencies are also transdiagnostic and visible in other mental disorders. Of course, autonomy deficiencies may be both a consequence of the disorder, but there is also evidence that these problems are already present before FND and psychopathology has developed. The autonomy-related variables we elaborate in this chapter are attachment, suggestibility, alexithymia, interoception, sense of agency, fear avoidance/openness to new experiences, and autonomy-connectedness. These factors have been scrutinized for the first time in recent years and provide initial evidence of autonomy deficiencies in FND.

3.1 Attachment in FND

Attachment in FND patients has also been studied more empirically only in recent years. Consequently, only a few studies are known. These do so far support an association between insecure attachment and FND. In clinical practice, we see that FND patients do not immediately see their problems in the light of problematic insecure attachment. They may see these problems as secondary to their symptoms. However, when we ask about past and present attachment relationships, it may become clear that patients have an inner working model that corresponds to problems with attachment. For example, patients mention that they have difficulty trusting themselves in relation to others or that they have difficulty making themselves dependent. Within partner relationships, problems are experienced during intimacy and patients are insecure and anxious in relation to others close to them. These problems often appear to have been present before the onset of FND symptoms, and this may mean that it is an important premorbid vulnerability factor. However, research that both before the pathology was present and after is still insufficient and should become an important area of research. Within FND, both avoidant attachment and anxious attachment have been demonstrated [13, 14] so far. In addition, it has also been shown that anxious attachment is associated with anxiety disorders and depression and also associated with alexithymia [15], which will be further explained below. In doing so, it appears that attachment affects the duration of FND-related symptoms [16]. Initial evidence that attachment may play a premorbid role is thus possibly explained.

In summary, there is evidence that there is an association between insecure attachment, alexithymia, and FND with other important related factors, such as depression and anxiety. Not enough longitudinal research has yet been done to make a statement about causality. Therefore, more research on attachment in FND needs to be done.

3.2 Suggestibility in FND

As earlier stated, probably one of the first persons to link the term suggestibility to FND (then called hysteria) was Martin Charcot around 1850 [1]. Although Charcot did not know how to explain this characteristic very well, he was able to characterize his patient population as 'suggestible.' Suggestibility refers to the capacity for suggestions to trigger automatized behavioral routines or mental representations and/or a tendency to form precise priors that override motor and perceptual systems [17]. Within the tradition, which we learned from historical literature [4], patients with 'hysteria' were treated, one of the first, by Freud and Breuer. Hypnotic suggestibility was a technique that was used. Breuer, in particular, believed in the hypnotic technique on which he could put patients under hypnosis and could expose patients in this way to traumatic effects. In this way, patients were able to integrate their effects and then become aware of feelings stored in their bodies. Those FND patients may be more susceptible to others' suggestions were later confirmed in various ways also in empirical research. For example, previous research shows that there is a significant association between hypnotic suggestibility and FND compared to a control group [18]. This may mean that patients are much more sensitive to what others think and adapt to it more quickly. This was also confirmed in a meta-analysis where the association between suggestibility and FND was systematically assessed [17]. The authors therefore argued that suggestibility makes patients more sensitive and susceptible to misinterpretation of body signals. It is suggested that dissociation also plays an important role in susceptibility to suggestion [17, 19]. This can be imagined when patients do not really know what they feel and therefore more likely to rely someone else's suggestions. So, hypnotic suggestibility and sensitivity to others' suggestions may play a role in maintaining FND and dissociative symptoms.

3.3 Alexithymia in FND

The disruption of emotional awareness, or alexithymia, refers to the incapability to have words for mood. By now, this topic is a well-known research topic that has been further empirically developed. It is sometimes put forward as an important premorbid factor for various forms of psychopathology, and especially psychosomatic problems [20]. An important assumption here is that patients did not get the words to the intersubjective emotions in their past lives from their important caregivers. Also, when there is too little mirroring and also emotional neglect, then patients have not been able to learn from their emotions. A study found a correlation between insecure attachment, depressive feelings, anxiety, and alexithymia within FND patients [15] as also earlier stated. This can mean that patients spiral into anxiety and gloom while at the same time not understanding what is going on inside them. The most common instrument still used to measure alexithymia is the TAS-20 (20-item Toronto Alexithymia Scale). The TAS-20 comprises three scales: difficulty identifying feelings, difficulty describing feelings, and externally oriented thinking. Externally oriented thinking refers to a thought process that is focused externally rather than internally. Internal orientation is a necessity for recognizing one's own feelings. However, the TAS-20 does not cover fantasizing conceived as another essential feature of alexithymia [21]. Therefore, it is necessary to investigate these factors of alexithymia also in FND in follow-up studies. Alexithymia is relatively common in FND and is estimated to be about 40% prevalent [22]. There is evidence that FND patients have difficulty identifying feelings and describing feelings [23]. However, too little is still known about which features of alexithymia are predominant in FND. In summary, there is evidence of an association between alexithymia and FND, but more research needs to be done to find out in what ways alexithymia plays a role.

3.4 Interoception in FND

Interoception includes how the nervous system experiences, interprets, and integrates signals from within the body. Interoception is believed to be a very important inner landscape that is considered a component of reflexes, urges, feelings, drives, adaptive responses, and cognitive and emotional experiences [24]. Interoception is a homeostatic feedback loop of the inner world—including the cardiovascular, pulmonary, gastrointestinal, genitourinary, nociceptive, chemosensory, osmotic, thermoregulatory, visceral, immune, and autonomic systems—on which people learn to trust and recognize what is experienced inside through reflections of the outer world [24]. This broad concept is difficult to operationalize because of its many aspects. A classification by Ricciardi et al. [25] works to operationalize three different facets of interoception in FND. For example, one can subdivide interoception into 'interoceptive accuracy' that refers to the accuracy of detecting bodily signals. In particular, this is operationalized by a heart rate task in which participants are asked to estimate their number of heartbeats. Here, it is assumed that if patients do not do very well, their degree of accuracy is limited. The second aspect refers to 'interoceptive sensibility' indicating a subjective report of one's ability to sense bodily signals that is operationalized with self-reported confidence questions such as the BAQ (Body Awareness Questionnaire). Examples of questions include 'I notice differences in the way my body reacts to various foods' and 'I am aware of a cycle in my activity level throughout the day' [26]. The third aspect includes 'interoceptive awareness' referring to the metacognitive awareness of one's interoceptive accuracy, usually calculated as the correspondence between accuracy and confidence. Recent results indicate that FND patients underperform on tasks measuring accuracy and sensitivity, but metacognitive aspects are intact [25]. This may mean that FND patients are aware of their inability of their interoceptive skills. Yet, these results are not uniform among FND patients. Indeed, other research shows no abnormalities in FND patients on accuracy, but does show abnormalities on sensibility [27]. Thus, although much research remains to be done on interoception in FND, there are initial indications of dysfunction in the area of sensibility among FND patients. Here, another interesting finding is that the increase in stress within this group does not matter much [14].

3.5 Sense of agency in FND

Sense of agency refers to the subjective experience of controlling our own thoughts and our bodily feelings. And, also important, it refers to a belief that self-generated action causes an event in the external environment. In movement disorders such as FND, this sense of agency process may be importantly affected [28]. A recent study shows that metabolic processes play a role in the decreased sense of agency of FND patients. This may also be related to patients' difficulty in reflecting on themselves [29]. This in turn is visible through disruptions within the so-called default network mode, a brain network, that is believed to be an important contributor to reflection, daydreaming, and spending time in the inner world. An important assumption here may be that FND patients experience deficits in their reflective functioning and where they may experience limited control over this. Although the sense of agency is a difficult construct to explore, there are increasing attempts to explore the construct further. Such is the case with FND. There are several ways in which the sense of agency has been measured in FND patients. For example, FMRI [30] has been used where there was support for a limitation of sense of agency in FND, and subliminal computer tasks have been experimented with in which no differences were found between non-psychiatric people and FND patients [31]. Yet, another research method that has been tried in FND patients is the rubber hand illusion task [32]. In the rubber hand illusion task, patients are watching the rubber hand tapping while performing tapping movements with their own fingers. To measure the sense of ownership and sense of agency, a questionnaire (mRHI) is used to examine statements such as 'I felt as if the rubber hand was my hand' (ownership statements) and 'I felt as if I caused the movement I saw' (agency statements). This suggests that patients with FND have more of an experience that the movements of the rubber hand match with the movements of their own hand; when in reality, this is not the case. Nevertheless, it appears that FND patients do not differ in their responses according to self-report results compared with controls [32].

In summary, the relevant construct 'sense of agency' is difficult to operationalize. This is evident in the various studies where researchers use different methods to measure the construct. This may play a role in the ambiguous results found so far in FND patients.

3.6 Fear avoidance/openness to new experience in FND

One broad theory that is further elaborated in developing psychopathology is the extent in which patients seek new situations. When people have a fear-avoiding temperament, this could lead to more inhibition and less novelty seeking and may contribute to psychopathology and less creativity [33]. FND patients may be more sensitive to negative information and may have difficulties seeking new situations [34]. 'More sensitivity to negative conditioning involves the progressive association of a neutral stimulus with fearful or negative outcomes, causing transference of negative saliency to the previous neutral stimulus' [34]. This is the behavioral explanation the authors suggested to illustrate how fear-avoidance sensitivity can lead to the conditioning of increased fear for new situations. This may explain why FND patients react with avoidance and dissociative strategies more than people within the normal population. There is some evidence to support this statement. For example, it has been shown that there is an association between low openness to new experiences and FND. Sarisoy et al. [35] found evidence to support the hypothesis that FND patients have lower novelty seeking and higher harm avoidance than control groups. This was measured by a self-report list used to measure temperament with the temperament and character inventory (TCI). The researchers hypothesized also that high harm avoidance, low reward dependency, low self-directedness, and high self-transcendence may be associated with dissociation and FND symptoms.

In summary, evidence suggests that openness to new experiences and harm avoidance may play a role in FND. Again, the evidence that has been found and the number of studies that have been done is limited making it difficult to link an obvious conclusion to the findings. However, it does raise interesting hypotheses about important premorbid factors of FND patients which we will now further translate into an integrated working model for FND patients which we will further discuss.

3.7 Autonomy-connectedness and a working model for FND patients

The concept of autonomy-connectedness may be a working model that integrates several premorbid autonomy-related personality variables. As shown above, there is initial evidence of correlation between premorbid autonomy-related personality factors and dissociative and FND symptoms [14, 15, 17]. The variables discussed earlier may be strongly related to deficiencies in autonomy-connectedness [12]. We will present an integrated working model that will now be the subject of more research and could possibly fit well with the problems of FND patients.

Central to autonomy-connectedness is the ability to be oneself and the ability to connect with others. Autonomy-connectedness refers to the need and capacity for separation and individuation and the need and capacity for intimacy and functioning in intimate relationships [36]. These two polarizing needs may be seen as a recurring dilemma that people may find themselves in. On the one hand, people want to belong, and, on the other hand, they want to be themselves. Being in contact with our own authentic bodily needs while staying connected with others is essential for our emotional and physical health. When people cannot connect enough with themselves, cut themselves off, and ignore bodily needs, it can lead to stress multiplication and may also lead to various physical ailments [37].

Autonomy-connectedness is embedded in the attachment theory [7, 9] which includes the conditions under which an infant can safely discover the world under the watchful eye of her caregivers and develop her autonomy under safe conditions. From this safety, infants increasingly become more autonomous by testing, extending, and then reducing their distance from their caregivers. Under this condition, infants can understand their own wants and needs separate from and in connection with their caregivers and others.

Autonomy-connectedness consists of three domains: first, self-awareness which contains the ability to be aware of opinions, wants, and needs and the ability to express these aspects of autonomy in social interactions. Second, sensitivity to others refers to sensitivity to the opinions, wants, and needs of others and the ability to empathize with others. Third, the ability to handle new situations which concerns how comfortable individuals are in situations that are not common.

Only recently has this theory been further developed at FND [38]. An elaborated hypothesis describes that FND patients have premorbid vulnerability before pathology develops. Moderating stressors such as interpersonal trauma, illness, grief, physical trauma, and work−/study-related problems may enhance the relationship between autonomy-connectedness deficits and FND-related symptoms. These symptoms can manifest at different levels such as interpersonal, intrapersonal, and biological. At the interpersonal level, patients may show high levels of self-sacrifice [39], and at the intrapersonal level, they articulate autonomy-connectedness conflicts. For example, 'on the one hand I want to live on my own, but on the other I don't dare.' At the biological level, this may result in hypoarousal.

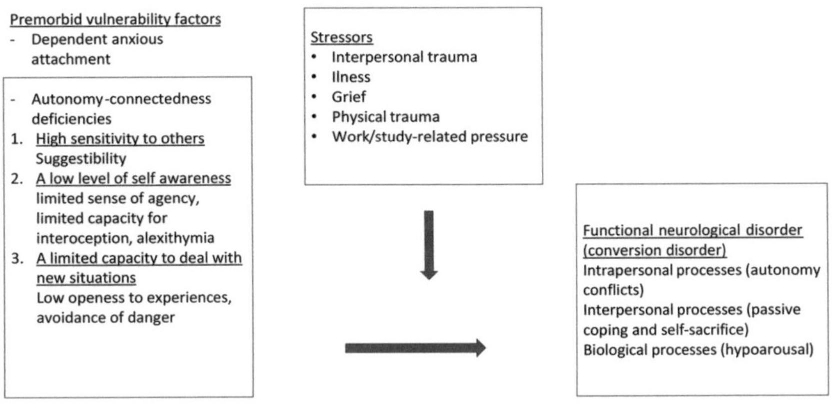

Figure 1.
A working model of autonomy-connectedness deficiencies in FND patients [38].

Hypoarousal is often related to the level of anxiety and depression [40]. Depression and anxiety disorders are often associated with FND (**Figure 1**) [41].

4. Treatment of autonomy in FND patients

Melanie is a patient with PNES symptoms that have been present for about two years. She described that her symptoms began at work. First, gradually, she could recognize in retrospect (not at the time) that she was becoming increasingly tired and experiencing mild dizziness that gradually got worse. Melanie worked within a hospital as a nurse and had worked her way up to a management position. As she gained this position, those around her noticed that she became increasingly direct and less friendly toward her colleagues. She explained that she needed to appear stronger and stronger. When Melanie was spoken to at work about her behavior, a short time later, an initial seizure occurred in which she fell off her chair and became unconscious. These attacks continued at work with fatigue, dizziness, and seizures eventually being classified by the neurologist as PNES. Melanie reports that, during a seizure, she can hear everything from her surroundings but is unable to respond. When Melanie talked about her past, she mentions that she never felt safe with her parents. The emphasis in her youth was always about strength and positivity. She was not allowed to whine in the face of adversity, and her mother denounced it when she could no longer hide her sadness when, for example, she was beaten by a classmate. According to her mother, she had to toughen herself up and stop being so 'pathetic.' This drama was repeated in her later relationships where Melanie was physically abused by her ex-partner who suffered from alcohol problems and had a short temper. Melanie mentions that she had to adapt to others very early on. She had to tiptoe around her parents and in later relationships to keep them from becoming angry with her. She never dared to think about her own physical and emotional signals, especially because these feelings were at odds with what those around her wanted from her. Melanie was always been anxious about seeking out new social situations. She was afraid of doing wrong to others. During the treatment, which focused on both psychological and psychomotor treatment, Melanie became aware of her autonomy-related problems. She recognized that she always looked at herself through someone else's eyes and had difficulty having her own views and opinions. She had doubts about who she was and what she wanted. Her emotions had no right to exist, and with every decision (even the smallest), she was wondering if this was the will of herself or the other. When Melanie became more aware of her own emotions and when she was able to admit them in relation to others (she now also has a partner whom she could trust), she could allow herself to develop her autonomy in relation to others. We got the impression that this could lead to a reduction in PNES-related symptoms and no longer played a meaningful role in her life.

This clinical example shows how a therapeutic process can be initiated after a patient is aware of her autonomy-related problems and can gradually learn to shape them differently. Becoming aware of problems that had been present in a patient's life for some time was an opening to develop a different narrative that is more focused on her own physical and emotional needs. This principle can be implemented within various therapeutic interventions.

There are different therapeutic 'techniques' that could be done for FND patients that are supportive for their autonomy. Think of the child who is repressed and rejected from the need for autonomy. Patients have often had the experience of having to adapt primarily and have not been seen in their needs to express themselves and gain experiences of direction and control. The question for therapy is How can patients increase their self-awareness a bit more again? Concepts such as those discussed earlier can help to clarify this. Patients have a limited ability to experience and describe and give language to what is happening inside them. Thus, they benefit from a therapeutic environment in which they can increase and integrate self-awareness.

An important question is whether this approach is so specific for patients with FND. An answer to this is that this is a transdiagnostic and person-oriented approach that is somewhat adapted to the underlying premorbid personality factors of patients with FND. Treatment can also be further specialized aimed at FND when physiotherapeutic, psychomotor, systemic, and psychological (such as catalepsy induction and medical hypnosis) interventions are used. However, it is expected that a therapeutic approach that focuses more on the underlying autonomy deficiencies and is integrated into a specific approach will be more durable and effective.

Author details

Luuk Stroink
Revalis Rehabilitation Centre, Nijmegen, Netherlands

*Address all correspondence to: luukstroink@hotmail.com

References

[1] Gilson F. Hysteria according to Charcot. The rise and disappearance of the 'nervous disorder of the century'; a medical historical study. Tijdschrift voor Psychiatrie. 2010;**52**:813-823

[2] Magnin E, Thomas-Antérion C, Sylvestre G, Haffen S, Magnin-Feysot V, Rumbach L. Conversion, dissociative amnesia, and Ganser syndrome in a case of "chameleon" syndrome: Anatomo-functional findings. Neurocase. 2014;**20**(1):27-36

[3] Ruesch J. The infantile personality: The core problem of psychosomatic medicine. Psychosomatic Medicine. 1948;**10**(3):134-144

[4] Freud S, Breuer J. Studies on Hysteria. Dutch Edition (1993). Klinische Beschouwingen, 5. Amsterdam: Boom; 1895

[5] Janet P. The mental state of hystericals. In: Robinson DN, editor. C.R. Corson (trans.), Significant Contributions to the History of Psychology, Series C, Medical Psychology, Vol. 11. Washington, DC: University Publications of America; 1977. (Original work published in 1982)

[6] Ludwig L, Pasman JA, Nicholson T, Aybek S, David AS, Tuck SEA. Stressful life events and maltreatment in conversion (functional neurological) disorder: Systematic review and meta-analysis of case-control studies. Lancet Psychiatry. 2018;**5**:307-320

[7] Blum HP. Separation-individuation theory and attachment theory. Journal of the American Psychoanalytic Association. 2004;**52**(2):535-553

[8] Muller J. Lacan's mirror stage. Psychoanalytic Inquiry. 1985;**5**(2):233-252

[9] Bowlby J. The Bowlby-Ainsworth attachment theory. Behavioral and Brain Sciences. 1979;**2**(4):637-638

[10] Ainsworth MDS. The Bowlby-Ainsworth attachment theory. Behavioral and Brain Sciences. 1978;**1**(3):436-438

[11] Steffen-Klatt A, Fiess J, Beckh J, Schmidt R, Rockstroh B. The impact of adverse childhood experience on symptom severity in patients with functional neurological symptom disorder (FNSD). Mental Health & Prevention. 2019;**13**:169-175

[12] Stroink L, Huijbregts K, Rakic A, Rijkeboer M, Bekker MH. The association between variables related to autonomy-connectedness and functional neurological disorders (FND): A systematic review. 2024. In preparation

[13] Cuoco S, Nisticò V, Cappiello A, Scannapieco S, Gambini O, Barone P, et al. Attachment styles, identification of feelings and psychiatric symptoms in functional neurological disorders. Journal of Psychosomatic Research. 2021;**147**:110539

[14] Williams IA, Reuber M, Levita L. Interoception and stress in patients with functional neurological symptom disorder. Cognitive Neuropsychiatry. 2021;**26**(2):75-94

[15] Williams B, Ospina JP, Jalilianhasanpour R, Fricchione GL, Perez DL. Fearful attachment linked to childhood abuse, alexithymia, and depression in motor functional neurological disorders. The Journal of Neuropsychiatry and Clinical Neurosciences. 2019;**31**(1):65-69

[16] Villagrán A, Lund C, Duncan R, Lossius MI. The effect of attachment

style on long-term outcomes in psychogenic nonepileptic seizures: Results from a prospective study. Epilepsy & Behavior. 2022;**135**:108890

[17] Wieder L, Brown R, Thompson T, Terhune DB. Suggestibility in functional neurological disorder: A meta-analysis. Journal of Neurology, Neurosurgery, and Psychiatry. 2021;**92**(2):150-157

[18] Roelofs K, Hoogduin KA, Keijsers GP, Näring GW, Moene FC, Sandijck P. Hypnotic susceptibility in patients with conversion disorder. Journal of Abnormal Psychology. 2002;**111**(2):390

[19] Wieder L, Terhune DB. Trauma and anxious attachment influence the relationship between suggestibility and dissociation: A moderated-moderation analysis. Cognitive Neuropsychiatry. 2019;**24**:191-207

[20] Lesser IM. A review of the alexithymia concept. Psychosomatic Medicine. 1981;**43**(6):531-543

[21] Bermond B, Oosterveld P, Vorst HCM. Measures of alexithymia. In: Boyle GJ, Saklofske DH, Matthews G, editors. Measures of Personality and Social Psychological Construct. London, UK: Academic Press; 2015. pp. 227-256

[22] Cole RH, Elmalem MS, Petrochilos P. Prevalence of autistic traits in functional neurological disorder and relationship to alexithymia and psychiatric comorbidity. Journal of the Neurological Sciences. 2023;**446**:120585

[23] Demartini B, Petrochilos P, Ricciardi L, Price G, Edwards MJ, Joyce E. The role of alexithymia in the development of functional motor symptoms (conversion disorder). Journal of Neurology, Neurosurgery & Psychiatry. 2014;**85**:1132-1137

[24] Khalsa SS, Adolphs R, Cameron OG, Critchley HD, Davenport PW, Feinstein JS, et al. Interoception and mental health: A roadmap. Biological Psychiatry: Cognitive Neuroscience and Neuroimaging. 2018;**3**(6):501-513

[25] Ricciardi L, Nisticò V, Andrenelli E, Cunha JM, Demartini B, Kirsch LP, et al. Exploring three levels of interoception in people with functional motor disorders. Parkinsonism & Related Disorders. 2021;**86**:15-18

[26] Shields SA, Mallory ME, Simon A. The body awareness questionnaire: Reliability and validity. Journal of Personality Assessment. 1989;**53**(4):802-815

[27] Millman LM, Short E, Stanton B, Winston JS, Nicholson TR, Mehta MA, et al. Interoception in functional motor symptoms and functional seizures: Preliminary evidence of intact accuracy alongside reduced insight and altered sensibility. Behaviour Research and Therapy. 2023;**168**:104379

[28] Seghezzi S, Convertino L, Zapparoli L. Sense of agency disturbances in movement disorders: A comprehensive review. Consciousness and Cognition. 2021;**96**:103228

[29] Charney M, Foster S, Shukla V, Zhao W, Jiang SH, Kozlowska K, et al. Neurometabolic alterations in children and adolescents with functional neurological disorder. NeuroImage: Clinical. 2024;**41**:103557

[30] Nahab FB, Kundu P, Maurer C, Shen Q, Hallett M. Impaired sense of agency in functional movement disorders: An fMRI study. PLoS One. 2017;**12**:e0172502

[31] Huys ACM, Edwards MJ, Bhatia KP, Haggard P. Modulation of reaction times and sense of agency via subliminal priming in functional movement

disorders. Frontiers in Neurology. 2020;**11**:989

[32] Marotta A, Bombieri F, Zampini M, Schena F, Dallocchio C, Fiorio M, et al. The moving rubber hand illusion reveals that explicit sense of agency for tapping movements is preserved in functional movement disorders. Frontiers in Human Neuroscience. 2017;**11**:291

[33] Baas M, Nijstad BA, Koen J, Boot NC, De Dreu CK. Vulnerability to psychopathology and creativity: The role of approach-avoidance motivation and novelty seeking. Psychology of Aesthetics, Creativity, and the Arts. 2020;**14**(3):334

[34] Morris LS, To B, Baek K, Chang-Webb YC, Mitchell S, Strelchuk D, et al. Disrupted avoidance learning in functional neurological disorder: Implications for harm avoidance theories. NeuroImage: Clinical. 2017;**16**:286-294

[35] Sarisoy G, Kaçar ÖF, Öztürk A, Yilman T, Mor S, Özturan DD, et al. Temperament and character traits in patients with conversion disorder and their relations with dissociation. Psychiatria Danubina. 2015;**27**(4):0-396

[36] Bekker MH. The development of an autonomy scale based on recent insights into gender identity. European Journal of Personality. 1993;7(3):177-194

[37] Maté G. When the Body Says No: Understanding the Stress-Disease Connection. Hoboken, New Jersey: John Wiley & Sons; 2011

[38] Stroink L, Huijbregts K. A reconsideration of premorbid factors in conversion disorders. Psychology and Psychotherapy Research Study. 2023;**7**(1):1-7

[39] Stroink L, Mens E, Ooms MH, Visser S. Maladaptive schemas of patients with functional neurological symptom disorder. Clinical Psychology & Psychotherapy. 2022;**29**(3):933-940

[40] Joiner TE Jr, Steer RA, Beck AT, Schmidt NB, Rudd MD, Catanzaro SJ. Physiological hyperarousal: Construct validity of a central aspect of the tripartite model of depression and anxiety. Journal of Abnormal Psychology. 1999;**108**(2):290

[41] Pehlivantürk B, Unal F. Conversion disorder in children and adolescents: A 4-year follow-up study. Journal of Psychosomatic Research. 2002;**52**:187-191

Chapter 3

Psychogenic Non-Epileptic Seizures: An Update on Diagnosis and Management

Sandro Misciagna

Abstract

Psychogenic non-epileptic seizures (PNES) are functional neurological disorders that mimic epileptic seizures. Over the past decades, relevant advancements have been made in the diagnosis, neurobiological understanding and management of PNES. This chapter is a review about epidemiology, comorbidities, biomarkers, neurobiology and treatment of PNES. The author discusses in particular the diagnosis of PNES that is based on clinical history, semiology, presence of witness and instrumental features. Neuroimaging studies suggest that PNES may occur in a context of anatomical alterations that regulate sensorimotor functions, emotional processing, cognitive control and multimodal integration of brain functions. The gold standard of PNES instrumental assessment remains video electroencephalography, showing the absence of epileptiform activity during the event and the absence of slow activity after the event. Several studies and clinical trials have demonstrated the importance of psychological treatments and in particular cognitive behavioral therapy. Further future studies are necessary to investigate about similarities and differences between psychogenic non-epileptic seizures, real epileptic seizures and other psychosomatic disorders. We also need studies for more appropriate psychotherapies and treatment guidelines.

Keywords: psychogenic non-epileptic seizures, conversion disorders, psychogenic seizures, dissociative seizures, pseudo-seizures, functional neurological disorders, PNES, cognitive behavioral therapy, psychotherapy, psychoeducational treatments

1. Introduction

Functional neurological disorders (FND) are common neurobehavioral conditions at the interface between neurology and psychiatry. Psychogenic non-epileptic seizures (or PNES) are a subtype of functional neurological disorder that consists of sudden and involuntary paroxysmal events characterized by disturbance in motor, autonomic, sensory, cognitive and emotional functions associated with alterations of consciousness and behavior. PNES frequently resemble epileptic seizures (ES) but are not associated with epileptic changes in cortical activity as demonstrated by EEG registrations [1].

Jean-Martin Charcot was one of the first neurologists to introduce PNES and other somatic symptoms in the medical literature as "hysteria." Subsequently, other researchers such as Sigmund Freud or Pierre Janet postulated psychological theories to explain this neurological condition [2]. In 1964, Liske and Foster created the term pseudo-seizures to refer to paroxysmal events similar to epileptic seizures but without EEG changes of epilepsy [3]. Over time, PNES received several names such as psychogenic seizures, pseudo-seizures, non-epileptic seizures, psychogenic non-epileptic attacks and psychogenic pseudo-seizures. Recently, other researchers have proposed to mention this condition as functional seizures [4] or dissociative seizures [5]. However, the most widely widespread term in current scientific literature is "psychogenic non-epileptic seizures" [6].

According to a modern vision, the conceptualization of PNES integrates both brain and mind [7].

Patients with PNES are often misdiagnosed for epilepsy and consequently treated with unnecessary antiepileptic drugs, emergency treatments and even hospital admissions.

Nowadays, notable advances have been made in the diagnosis and treatment of patients with PNES. Epidemiology studies have demonstrated that the treatment of patients with PNES needs a comprehensive multidisciplinary approach. Advances in clinical neuroscience are starting to better understand etiology, neurobiology, pathophysiological mechanisms and biomarkers of PNES. This coud facilitate the diagnosis and treatment. This chapter is a review about PNES focusing in particular on diagnostic criteria, semiological features that distinguish PNES from epileptic seizures and evidence-based treatment interventions.

2. Epidemiology

Psychogenic non-epileptic seizures is a neurobehavioral condition that occurs worldwide with a prevalence of approximately 1.5% per 100,000 inhabitants per year [8]. However, epidemiological data on PNES are limited and sparse. A study conducted in Iceland estimated the incidence of PNES as 1.4 per 100.000, with symptoms commonly emerging from 20 to 40 years [9]. Studies conducted in the USA have demonstrated that up to 20% of civilians and up to 25% of veterans diagnosed as epileptic, on the contrary, have PNES [10]. Therefore, PNES is common as other neurological diseases such as Parkinson's disease or multiple sclerosis [11]. Epidemiological investigations conducted in Ohio have estimated prevalence of PNES up to 33/100,000 individuals [9], while prospective studies conducted on 367,566 individuals followed for 3 years found an incidence rate of 4.9/100,000 per year [12].

Regarding gender differences, PNES individuals are typically women in approximately 80% of cases, with a mean age of onset of 31 years ± 15 years. Prevalence is higher in women, probably due to social and neurobiological differences [13].

The majority of PNES patients are unemployed, 43% received a prior diagnosis with depression or anxiety, and 57% had at least one medically unexplained symptom [14]. Even if PNES can be detected at any age and can have many stereotypes, younger women with high levels of mental health and a history of past abuse are more likely to be among the patient group. The coincidence of PNES with epileptic seizures is about 10% [15]. Epilepsy may also increase the risk of PNES through biological mechanisms and by experiencing epileptic seizures [16].

3. Comorbidities and risk factors

Adult patients with PNES have various comorbid medical, neurological and psychiatric conditions that contribute to prognosis and treatment responses. A two-year retrospective review on 158 patients with PNES demonstrated that they were more likely to report a history of other medical conditions and in particular somatic syndromes such as chronic fatigue syndrome, fibromyalgia, chronic pain and irritable bowel syndrome [17]. These patients also often suffer from chronic, intermittent medical conditions such as asthma and migraine [17]. When compared with ES with the use of medical questionnaires, PNES patients frequently report a history of traumatic brain injury or have comorbidity with intellectual disabilities [15].

Psychiatric disorders that may be found in comorbidity with PNES are affective disorders [18], anxiety, depression, eating disorders [19] and other somatoform disorders [7], but also personality disorders, in particular clusters B and C of personality disorders [20].

Another psychiatric disorder often associated with PNES is post-traumatic stress disorder (PTSD). In fact, three-fourths of individuals with PNES report traumatic experiences including physical abuses (in about 25% of cases) or sexual abuses (in about 30% of cases) [21]. Patients with a history of sexual abuses exhibit an earlier event onset, more severe convulsions, emotional disorders and other post-traumatic symptoms [22]. Patients with eating disorders often have a history of prior trauma and subsequent PTSD and related psychiatric comorbidities [19]. Individuals with prior traumas are more likely to have comorbid psychiatric conditions and dissociative symptoms [23]. Studies on the association between PNES and PTSD have been conducted in retrospective reviews of veterans with PNES and 37 veterans with ES. These studies have demonstrated that PTSD symptoms preceded the diagnosis of PNES in 58% of patients and that PTSD comorbidity was able to differentiate between PNES and ES [10]. Veterans with PNES showed more non-motor or hypomotor PNES events [24].

Patients with PNES have abnormal neuropsychiatric and personality profiles. Depressive symptoms are associated with PNES even if depression scores on psychometric questionnaires do not differentiate between PNES and ES [25].

Patients with PNES can also have dissociative symptoms such as fragmentation of internal experience of the outside world (derealization) or fragmentation of perception of body schema (depersonalization) linked to somatic symptoms and depression [26]. Alexithimia that consists in the reduced ability to express and recognize emotions, has also been observed in PNES patients. However, it is not clear if alexithimia scores can differentiate between PNES and ES [27].

Studies based on cluster analysis suggest that patients with PNES could have different subtypes of psychopathologies. For example, in a cohort study of 43 PNES subjects, 11 individuals were categorized as having high levels of psychopathologic disorders with somatization, alexithimia and impairment in emotional regulation, while 32 individuals were categorized as having high levels of somatization disorders and depression, but relatively normal emotion expression [28].

Personality of subjects with PNES has been studied with psychiatric instruments such as Minnesota Multiphasic Personality Inventory (MMPI-2) or Personality Assessment Inventory (PAI). In a cohort of 75 patients with PNES and 109 patients with ES, Personality Assessment Inventory showed significant high scores in somatic, conversion, anxious, depression and suicidal symptoms [29]. Instead, Minnesota Multiphasic Personality Inventory showed a "conversion V pattern" with elevation in hypochondria and hysteria in depression subscales [30]. Regression analysis suggests that the use of health scales and conversion scales of PAI and hysteria subscale of MMPI2 could be useful to distinct between PNES and ES patients [31].

Neuropsychological studies have not demonstrated different cognitive profile of PNES patients when compared to ES patients. However, PNES subjects frequently complain cognitive symptoms including concentration difficulties and memory disorders. Cognitive studies have demonstrated that PNES patients potentially overestimate their cognitive deficits. In neuropsychological assessment, they have generally worse performance in tests that consist in word finding and some specific language tests such as Boston Naming Test [32]. Other studies have demonstrated that patients with PNES show some impairment in tests that explore attention, executive functions, spatial working memory [33] or difficulty in switching attention from emotion-related task demands [34]. A study conducted on patients with PNES and a story of prior trauma and patients with PNES without prior trauma showed that patients with PNES and PTSD had lower performances in neuropsychological tests exploring verbal memory performances than the group of patients without PTSD [35].

Numerous studies identified potential risk factors, precipitant factors and perpetuating factors for PNES. As already mentioned, predisposing factors for PNES are generally traumatic experiences such as physical or sexual abuses since they increase the vulnerability of the subjects [16]. Precipitating factors that trigger PNES attacks are generally stressor situations such as death or separation events (such as death of a friend or a family member, and job loss), natural disasters or relationship difficulties, since they occur before the onset of the attacks [36]. Perpetuating factors of PNES are psychological comorbidities such as mood disorders (anxiety, depression), anger and mistreatments [16].

4. Neurological diagnosis of PNES

When a medical doctor tries to reach the diagnosis of a PNES, it is important to consider that about 10% of patients with psychogenic non-epileptic seizures have also epilepsy [37]. PNES must be distinguished from other disorders such as sleep disorders, migraine, syncope, movement disorders and transient ischemic attacks that are mediated by other pathophysiological mechanisms [13].

Approaches for diagnosis of PNES include clinical history, symptom provocation, observation and EEG analysis [36]. Characteristic historical features and semiologic signs [38] that help to distinguish PNES from epileptic attacks are listed in **Table 1**.

Clinical signs evaluated to distinguish between PNES and seizures consist in motor, somatic and other signs. Motor signs have been reported in controlled studies where a video-EEG was used to diagnose the events. Examples of motor signs that can help to differentiate PNES from seizures are long duration of the event, a fluctuating course, the presence of asynchronous movements, pelvic thrusting, side-to-side head movements, ictal eye closure at onset, ictal crying and post-ictal recall of information. However, there are no pathognomonic signs that totally rule out epileptic seizures [39]. For example, non-synchronic hypermotor symptoms that were considered typical of PNES are not specific since they could be seen in epileptic seizures originated in frontal lobe or in generalized tonic-clonic seizures [40]. Moreover, between 8 and 31% of patients with PNES have suffered injuries during seizures such as tongue biting, bumps and falls [41]. Urinary incontinence [42] and appearance

Historical features	PNES	Epileptic seizures
Associated psychiatric disorders	One or multiple	Generally absent
Prior sexual or physical abuses	In about 30% of cases	Absent
Intellectual disability	Frequent	In encephalopathies
Emergency department visits	Multiple	Occasional
Seizure frequency	High	Variable
Injury from seizures	Absent	Occasional
Response to antiepileptic	Absent	Up to 70% of cases
Experience with epilepsy	Frequent in family	In genetic forms
Setting of seizures	Generally in the presence of others	Variable
Semiological features	PNES	Epileptic seizures
Emotional triggers	Present	Absent
Onset of the event	Gradual	Sudden
Duration of the event	Long duration	Short duration
Progression	Fluctuating course	Physiological course
Symptomatology	Variable	Stereotyped
Ictal crying	Usually present	Usually absent
Movements during the event	Asynchronous	Synchronous
Breathing during the event	Normal	Stertorous
Eyes closure during the event	Forced	Not forced
Anxiety during the attack	Present	Absent
Autonomic signs	Common	Infrequent
Kind of tongue biting	Not on the side	On the side
Post-ictal confusion	Absent	Present
Memory of the event	Present	Absent

Table 1.
Main historical and semiologic differences between psychogenic non-epileptic seizures (PNES) and epileptic seizures (ES).

of seizures during sleep [43] have been also described in patients with PNES even if they are more frequent in epilepsy. On the other hand, post-ictal confusion supports the diagnosis of epileptic seizures. Post-ictal stertorous breathing supports diagnosis of epileptic seizure, but only in cases of convulsive events. In events that resemble syncope, a sudden collapse to the ground with eyes closed for more than 2 minutes is characteristic of psychogenic non-epileptic events. Other useful clinical signs proposed for diagnosis of PNES are: ictal stuttering [44] and the bringing of an inappropriate toy animal during video-EEG monitoring (known as teddy bear sign) which has a specificity of 100% but a sensitivity between 5.2 and 9% [45].

Somatic signs of anxiety during the attacks are more frequent in PNES compared to epileptic seizures and can help in the diagnosis [46]. The presence during or after a panic attack at least 4 of the 13 symptoms of anxiety reported in DSM-4 TR has a sensitivity of 83% and specificity of 65% [47]. These symptoms include: (1) palpitations or pounding heart, (2) sweating, (3) trembling or shaking, (4) sensation of shortness, (5) feeling of choking, (6) chest pain, (7) nausea or abdominal distress, (8) dizziness, (9) derealization or depersonalization, (10) fear of losing control, (11) fear of dying, (12) paresthesia and (13) chills or hot flushes [48]. Other relatively common signs that support the diagnosis of a PNES are: gradual onset, the presence of non-stereotyped movements, thrashing movements, opisthotonos and tongue biting [49].

Patients with PNES can have impaired state of conscience such as lack of responsiveness, psychic symptoms, aura that may resemble generalized absence seizures or temporal seizures with automatisms [50]. Other types of PNES such as psychogenic atonic seizures or presyncopes may show behavioral arrest, immobility, psychic aura, unusual somatic sensations, dissociation states (derealization and depersonalization) and hallucinations (auditory, visual and olfactory) resembling seizures with impaired state of conscience [51]. In patients with PNES, autonomic manifestations are also common such as tachycardia, incontinence, flushing and sweating [46]. Specific triggers such as flashing lights could provoke attacks of PNES, while intermittent light stimulation is observed in some forms of photo-inducted epileptic syndromes [46]. Other elements are characteristic of PNES; for example, patients with PNES are more likely to have attacks in the presence of others or in medical settings [38] or can talk about the attacks since have memory of the event [52].

Even if clinical signs are useful for the diagnosis of PNES, instrumental features are useful [53].

One of the most important instrumental examinations that differentiates PNES from real seizures is based on the use of standard electroencephalography. Typical events of PNES are characterized by lack of electrographic changes [54], while an EEG with epileptic anomalies followed by slow abnormalities and sleep supports the diagnosis of epileptic seizures.

Gold standard for the diagnosis of PNES is video-EEG monitoring and recording of positive EEG features during the episodes [55]. Video-EEG consists in the continuous monitoring of patient's behavior during the paroxysmal episodes, while electrical brain activity is simultaneously recorded through the surface electrodes of the EEG [56]. Video-EEG monitoring is a highly specific and sensitive technique with a diagnostic yield of 50 to 60 percent. Video-EEG could not be available and some patients may have low event frequencies so that admission for long-term EEG monitoring is impractical. The absence of video-EEG recording can result in false-positive diagnosis [57]. A perspective study has shown that epileptic seizures are misdiagnosed as PNES more likely than the opposite with a frequency of 57 vs. 12% [58]. Furthermore, epileptic seizures of fronto-mesial origin are often misdiagnosed as PNES since semiology can mimic a pseudo-seizure and EEG often fails to identify ictal patterns [43].

Recently, using a combination of history, witness description and clinical signs, and EEG findings, the International League Against Epilepsy (ILAE) Commission on Neuropsychobiology Non-Epileptic Seizure Task Force has published a consensus guideline on the minimal criteria to diagnosis of PNES. According to ILAE, "Documented PNES" criteria consists in clinical history in favor of PNES and confirmation with video-EEG demonstrating the absence of epileptiform activity. Lower levels of certainly depend on availability of diagnostic components (see **Table 2**).

Given the need to clarify a diagnosis of PNES, whenever possible, the use of provocation EEG techniques including hyperventilation and photic stimulation may be effective procedures [59]. Standard induction protocols may aid diagnostic

DOI: http://dx.doi.org/10.5772/intechopen.1005425

Diagnostic level	History	Witness event	EEG finding
Possible PNES	+	Self-reported and/or witness description	Absence of epileptiform activity in routine EEG or sleep-deprived interictal EEG
Probable PNES	+	Physicians witnessed the event or reviewed a video showing typical semiological findings of PNES	Absence of epileptiform activity in routine EEG or sleep-deprived interictal EEG
Clinically established PNES	+	Clinical experienced in epilepsy reviewed the video or witnessed an event showing semiology, while not on EEG typical of PNES	Absence of epileptiform activity in routine EEG or sleep-deprived EEG registered during an equivalent epileptic seizure
Documented PNES	+	Clinical experienced in diagnosis of epilepsy reviewed the video or witnessed an event showing semiology typical of PNES	Absence of epileptiform activity in EEG registered immediately before, during and after the event captured by video-EEG

Table 2.
Diagnostic levels of PNES according to ILAE.

evaluation. Surface electromyography recordings could also help to differentiate PNES from convulsive epileptic seizures events [60].

5. Psychiatric diagnosis of PNES

There are different psychiatric categories that represent the so-called PNES.

According to the Diagnostic and Statistical Manual of Mental Disorders, version 4 Text Revision (DSM-4 TR), PNES with motor disorders are mainly represented by the category of somatoform disorders [48]. According to this classification, somatoform disorders are subdivided into four categories: conversion disorders with motor symptoms, conversion disorders with sensory symptoms, conversion disorders with seizures and conversion disorders with mixed presentation. However, when an impairment of conscience is evident, PNES could be better represented by the category of dissociative disorders.

The Diagnostic and Statistical Manual of Mental Disorders, version 5 (DSM-5) has replaced conversion and dissociative categories in functional neurological disorders, which encompasses all types of PNES [61]. According to this classification, PNES disorders would be considered as functional rather than structural disturbances of central nervous system.

According to the 10th version of the International Classification of Diseases (ICD-10), conversion disorders include the categories of conversion hysteria, conversion reaction, hysterical psychosis and dissociative seizures [62]. Therefore, ICD-10 considers PNES within mental and behavioral disorders that are somatoform and dissociative disorders. Dissociative disorders are characterized by alteration of normal integration between memories of the past, awareness of own identity and sensation of loss of control of body movements.

According to the 11th version of the International Classification of Diseases (ICD-11), dissociative disorders are considered in a separate way by somatic symptoms in the chapter about mental, behavioral and neurodevelopmental disorders. The ICD-11 classifies conversion disorders as neurotic, somatoform and stress-related disorders [63].

6. Rating scales for PNES

Cianci et al. in 2011 developed a rating scale for psychogenic non-epileptic seizures PNES [64] (See **Table 3**).

For this purpose, 60 PNES patients were included in the study. These patients had EEG without ictal or interictal epileptiform activity and no post-ictal slowing. The rating scale showed a high sensitivity, specificity and inter-rater reliability that ranged from 0.69 to 1 in case of the presence or absence of motor signs and associated features [65]. In a study that compared this scale to the Clinical Global Impression (CGI), a non-specific scale, researchers demonstrated a strong correlation (with a Spearman correlation score of 0.69) between the mean CGI score and the total PNES score. The limitations of the PNES scale are such as the ability to evaluate the severity of the event or clearly define the associated events that support the diagnosis of PNES. Finally, this scale gives more importance to motor phenomena rather than the assessment of consciousness.

Further studies are necessary to clarify the relationship between PNES, cognitive deficits and anxiety and mood symptoms to understand in particular if these deficits occur independently.

7. Biomarkers

Since EEG is not available in many centers, researches have studied various substances as potential biomarkers for differentiation between PNES and epileptic seizures.

According to many studies, serum creatine phosphokinase (CPK) levels should be able to differentiate epileptic seizures from PNES with a sensitivity of 75% and a specificity of 85.5% [66, 67]. In different studies, serum creatine phosphokinase correlates positively with occurrence of real seizures, while none of patients with PNES show elevation in serum levels of CPK [68].

Some pituitary hormones such as prolactin (PRL), thyrotropin-releasing hormone (TRH) and growth hormone (GH) have resulted increased in serum following epileptic seizures but not in PNES [68, 69]. For example, a study demonstrated that 10-20 minutes following an ictal event, prolactin levels were approximately doubled in the serum of epileptic patients but not in PNES patients [70–72].

Scale for motor phenomena				**Scale for associated features**	
Motor phenomena	**Presence**	**Severity**	**Duration**	**Associated features**	**Presence**
Tonic tremor Clonic tremor Hypermotor/agitation Atonic/akinetic Automatisms	0 = absent 1 = present	0 = none 1 = minimal 2 = mild 3 = moderate 4 = severe	0 = none 1 = <25% of the time 2 = 25–50% of the time 3 = 50–75% of the time 4= > 75% of the time	Incontinence Tongue biting Drooling Eye closure Hyperventilation Lament/crying	0 = absent 1 = present

Table 3.
Rating scale for PNES.

Results related to cortisol level are controversial. Some authors have demonstrated pre-ictal decrease and post-ictal increase of cortisol in epileptic patients and no changes in PNES patients [73]. Other studies showed basal hypercorticolism in PNES patients and a positive correlation with both levels of vigilance, traumatic history [74] and attentional difficulties in an emotional Stroop task [75]. Some authors speculated that PNES patients have hyperactivation of hypothalamic-pituitary axis (HPA axis); then, adrenocorticotropic hormone (ACTH) is hyper-secreted into blood stream and induces release of cortisol. In fact, as mentioned previously, nearly 50% of PNES patients have psychological disorders related to trauma or post-traumatic stress disorders [76]. Therefore, stress response would induce activation of sympathetic nervous system (SNS) and hypothalamic-pituitary axis resulting in increased cortisol levels. The activation of SNS and HPA axis could also led to health consequences such as growth disorders or autoimmune diseases [77]. Other changes in potential biomarkers have been attributed to stress problems in PNES patients such as high levels of testosterone and lower levels of oxytocina in women with a history of chronic stress or childhood abuse [78]. Instead, estradiol level is lower in women with stressful conditions [79].

Other hormonal biomarkers have been studied as diagnostic tools for PNES such as nesfatin, ghrelin and brain-derived neurotrophic factors (BDNF) [80]. Serum and salivary levels of nesfatin were found to be high in post-ictal epileptic seizures compared to PNES [81]. Instead, post-ictal serum ghrelin levels were lower in patients who had epileptic seizures if compared to ones who had PNES [82]. Brain-derived neurotrophic factors are neurotrophins implicated in neurogenesis and synaptic reorganization. BDNF have resulted reduced in a sample of PNES patients compared to healthy controls [83] or in patients with depressive disorders [84]. However, post-ictal levels of BDNF resulted similar in ES and PNES patients; therefore, BDNF is not a biomarker specific in differentiating seizure types. This happens since BDNF levels are probably related to stress than to seizure type [76].

Neuropeptide Y (NPY), an inhibitory neuromodulator of the brain that could control propagation of limbic seizures, has been studied in epileptic and PNES patients. The presence of stress disorders could help to reduce the levels of NPY and determine the onset of PNES symptoms. In fact, different studies have demonstrated lower level of NPY in PNES patients in comparison with healthy subjects [85].

Finally, PNES patients have post-ictal higher levels of a natriuretic peptide hormone called C-type natriuretic peptide (CNP) that is a hormone produced by nervous system cells as well as by endothelial cells and bone cells [86]. Authors hypothesized that the difference is due to increased blood-brain barrier permeability, synaptic stabilization and altered microcirculation [87].

8. Neurobiology and pathophysiology of PNES

Structural neuroimaging studies have started to understand neurobiology of PNES [7]. Techniques based on the use of functional magnetic resonance imaging (f-MRI) and positron emission tomography (PET) have tried to investigate neural functional connectivity anomalies in PNES [88, 89]. On the bases of these studies, researchers have demonstrated that PNES patients have an increased functional connectivity between motor regions localized in precentral sulcus and regions involved in emotional processing localized in anterior cingulate cortex or regions involved in frontal function (such as executive functions) localized in inferior frontal gyrus and parietal cortex [90]. Instead, other studies have found functional connectivity dissociation between the precentral sulcus and the posterior insula [89]. Several neuroanatomical studies have demonstrated functional connectivity alterations in networks implicated in executive and attentional functions, emotional control and sensorimotor functions [91]. Other research that had the purpose to study functional connectivity patterns in PNES patients compared to healthy subjects demonstrated increased functional connectivity between left ventral anterior insula, left post-central gyrus and bilateral supplementary motor area [92]. Functional connectivity between the bilateral supplementary motor areas positively correlated with the frequency of psychogenic seizures [93]. Functional connectivity between supplementary motor areas and anterior cingulate cortex also positively correlated with the frequency of psychogenic seizures [92]. A PET study that compared cerebral metabolism between healthy subjects and patients with PNES demonstrated that patients with psychogenic non-epileptic seizures had hypometabolism in bilateral anterior cingulate cortex and right inferior parietal lobule [88].

Neuroimaging studies based on the use of quantitative structural MRI and voxel-based morphometry (VBM) have demonstrated that patients with PNES have anterior cingulate cortex, supplementary motor areas and pre- and post-central gyrus atrophy [94]. Other studies showed reduction in the thickness of the cortex in insular and orbitofrontal regions in PNES patients [95].

A diffusion tensor tractography (DTT) study that compared PNES patients to healthy subjects demonstrated in PNES patients a right asymmetry of the uncinated fasciculus, which is a tract that connects medial prefrontal cortex with medial temporal regions [96].

All these anatomical and functional neuroimaging studies suggest that PNES patients have a context of cerebral alterations that concern interactions across brain areas designated to sensorimotor functions, cognitive control, emotion processing and multimodal integration. Further research is necessary to confirm these findings and better understand neural circuit alterations and cerebral network dysfunctions. Researchers should also study better neurofunctional circuit alterations in specific psychiatric functional patter or semiological frameworks such as convulsive vs. atonic events.

Autonomic nervous system studies and electrophysiological studies are also contributing to understand pathophysiology of non-epileptic psychogenic seizures. For example, a study based on EEG analyses conducted in a cohort or 18 PNES patients and 18 health control subjects, demonstrated a reduction of functional connectivity between basal ganglia and cortical regions and a reduction of interhemispheric connectivity across paralimbic areas [97]. Some autonomic investigations have demonstrated an increase in sympathetic tone ictally in epileptic seizures rather than non-epileptic psychogenic seizures [98], while other studies have documented pre-ictal and post-ictal autonomic changes between the two groups [99].

9. Treatment of PNES

PNES is a condition that causes social stigma for both patients and their families. The understanding of the factors determining the psychogenic non-epileptic seizures is important to predict the patient's response to the diagnosis and subsequent therapies.

To the present days, significant progresses have been made in the management of PNES [71]. The management of PNES can be divided in four phases. The first phase (diagnostic phase) aims to communicate the diagnosis of PNES to the patients who are often confused and irritated. The second phase (engagement phase) consists in making the patients aware of the diagnosis and make them actively participating to the treatments. The third phase (acute intervention phase) aims to reduce the frequency of seizures, improve psychiatric comorbidities and improve quality of life. The fourth phase (long-term intervention) aims to manage in the long-term PNES patients. A pioneering study conducted in 1998 demonstrated that a clear explanation of PNES diagnosis, combined with immediate psychological treatment, markedly reduces the use of medical services [100]. How the diagnosis is communicated is very important since a correct information to the patient and his family about non-epileptic origin of the seizures can remit the symptoms in some patients [101] or can have consequences on the evolution of the seizures [102]. After the diagnosis of PNES, the treating neurologist gradually discontinues antiepileptic medications and simultaneously starts other specific treatments.

The best strategies of treatment for PNES are psychotherapies, psychotropic medications or other psychiatric interventions based on evidence that PNES patients have a huge variety of psychological and psychiatric disorders [103]. Clinicians have proposed a wide variety of psychotherapeutically interventions that include cognitive behavioral approaches, psychodynamic interpersonal therapy, mindfulness-based therapies, psychoeducational therapy, group and family therapies, psychodynamic therapies, supportive psychotherapy and hypnosis [18].

Cognitive behavioral therapy (CBT) is one of the most useful approaches to a wide range of clinical and psychological factors. Cognitive behavioral therapy has a proven effectiveness for treatment of anxiety and depression, frequently associated with development and maintenance of PNES [104]. In a randomized trial of 12 weeks conducted on 66 patients with PNES, CBT associated with standard medical care showed a statistically significant reduction in seizure frequency at the end of the treatment sessions [105]. Goldstein proposed a 12-session model focused on cognitive, emotional and behavioral aspects of PNES [105]. According to this model, the treatment consists in five stages. The first stage consists in commitment to treatment and rational explanation. The second stage is teaching techniques for controlling pseudo-seizures. The third stage is exposing techniques to reduce avoidance. The fourth stage is the management of emotions and cognition related to seizures. The last stage is relapse prevention [105].

Howlet and Reuber have developed a brief psychodynamic interpersonal therapy (PDIT) for the treatment of patients with PNES (Howlet and [106]). They proposed an empathetic approach aimed to improve copying stiles and promote patient collaboration. Treatment consists of an initial two-hour semi-structured interview followed by 19 therapy sessions with intervals of 1 or 2 weeks. A study conducted on 108 patients with PNES treated with this model demonstrated that between 12 and 60 months after the end of the therapy, 40% of patients presented a 50% reduction of pseudo-seizures and 25% of patients were seizure free [107].

Mindfulness-based therapies (MBT) try to promote self-regulation of attention, adopt an attitude of curiosity and accept own experience at each moment. According to Baslet, MBT program is organized in five modules that include psychoeducation, mindfulness for everyday life, stress management strategies, emotion management and relapse prevention [107]. In PNES patients, MDT determined reduction in the seizure frequency and improvement in quality of life.

Acceptance commitment therapy (ACT) is a hybrid psychotherapy with components derived from both cognitive behavior therapy and mindfulness-based therapy [108]. ACT has demonstrated efficacy in the treatment of depression, post-traumatic stress disorder, dissociative conditions and experimentally in psychogenic seizures [109]. It focuses on enhancing individual psychological flexibility using techniques that changes patient's relationship with his own emotions. In a study conducted on a small group of patients, ACT showed clinically significant improvement in psychological flexibility and reduction in seizure episodes [110].

Approaches based on psychoeducational programs (PEP) have been demonstrated to be important in the management of patients with PNES. The basis of this treatment consists in making the patient aware of his condition through the use of educational modules aimed to explain psychogenic origin of seizures and treating the associated aspects. PEP are mainly designed in a group format. One of the first PEP was proposed by Zaroff in USA in 2004 who reported improvement in post-traumatic symptoms, dissociation and perceived quality of life [111]. A randomized controlled trial conducted by Chen on PNES patients showed that psychoeducational intervention improves psychosocial functioning and reduces access to emergency rooms, visits and hospitalizations, but if it does not reduce frequency and intensity of PNES [112]. Other studies based on psychoeducational treatment that included among the interventions explanation regarding mind-body relationship, distraction exercises and relaxation have determined also a significant decrease in the frequency of PNES [113].

Some researchers have proposed group and family therapies (GFT) in patients with PNES since their families are more conflictive than those of epileptic patients [114]. These therapies have demonstrated improvement in psychological well-being but variable results regarding the reduction of seizures [115].

Psychodynamic therapies (PDT) are based on the psychoanalytic concept of trauma using principles of Anna Freud's psychology and object relations theory. A study conducted by de Olivera Santos applying psychodynamic therapy reported a 30% of seizure-freedom in patients with PNES [116].

Other studies have reported that prolonged exposure therapy (PET) reduces the number of PNES and improves post-traumatic symptomatology for patients diagnosed with PNES and PTSD [117]. For example, a study conducted on 16 patients diagnosed with PNES and PTSD, after 12–15 weekly sessions they had a significant reduction in seizure frequency and PTSD symptoms and maintained these improvements for a long period [118].

In recent years, eye movement desensitization and reprocessing (EMDR) has also been proposed in the treatment pf patients diagnosed with PNES and post-traumatic stress disorders [119]. However, it has not shown effective results when used as first line of treatment and it is more useful if associated with a battery of treatments [106].

In addition to psychotherapeutically interventions, when depression or post-traumatic stress disorders are present in comorbidity, some antidepressant drugs are effective as pharmacological treatment. Serotonin reuptake inhibitors (SSRI) are the antidepressants with more effective results. For example, a double-blind, randomized, placebo-controlled study conducted over 12 weeks showed that sertraline treatment determined a reduction of 45% of seizure frequency; instead, placebo treatment determined an increase of 8% of seizure frequency [120]. A multicenter randomized clinical trial conducted in 2014 compared four types of treatment: only sertraline with a flexible dose, only cognitive behavioral psychotherapy, association of sertraline with CBT and standard medical care [121]. This study demonstrated that the two groups that received psychotherapy exhibited a significant reduction in seizures: 51% in the group treated only with cognitive behavioral psychotherapy and 59% in the group treated with association of sertraline with CBT. The group of patients treated with standard medical care did not show a significant reduction in the frequency of seizures. The group treated only with cognitive behavioral psychotherapy showed improvement in many psychological disorders such as anxiety, depression and global functioning. These findings support that in patients with non-epileptic seizures, it is possible to control the seizures with an approach based on use of psychotherapies and in particular cognitive behavioral therapy [122].

Long-term benefits of therapies have been examined in randomized controlled clinical trials that take in consideration pharmacologic and psychotherapy options of intervention [123].

Outcomes of PNES subjects are improved when the assessment of these patients is based on accurate diagnosis, effective communication with the patient and correct management [124]. A retrospective study of 260 consecutive PNES patients measuring outcome at six and 12 months after diagnosis demonstrated that 18% showed an increase in seizures, 38% were seizures free and the majority of patients continued to have seizures [125]. Patients with psychiatric disorders such as anxiety or depression had less chances to become seizure free. In addition to psychiatric and psychosocial disorders, patients with PNES and a story of traumatic brain injury have worse outcomes other than increased depression, impulsivity, behavioral disorders and lower global functioning [72].

10. Conclusions

Psychogenic non-epileptic seizures are functional neurologic disorders with high prevalence. In recent years, relevant advancement has been made in diagnosis and the management of this neuropsychiatric condition. Accurate diagnosis and management of PNES need a multidisciplinary collaborative approach among neurologists, psychiatrists and other specialists. In addition to an accurate medical history, research for clinical signs and video-EEG, different biomarkers could help the diagnosis of PNES. Examples of biomarkers useful for differentiating PNES from epileptic seizures are hyper-cortisolism, delayed creatine phosphokinase, lower post-ictal levels of nesfatin and elevated post-ictal levels of ghrelin. Neuroimaging studies are helping clinicians to clarify neurobiology of PNES and reduce the stigma associated with this condition. Although there is a general agreement that psychogenic non-epileptic seizures can be treated with psychotherapies, the effectiveness of the most psychotherapeutic methods has not been adequately investigated. Future investigations will be useful to identify new biomarkers and psychopathological mechanism for an appropriate diagnosis and treatment of PNES.

Conflict of interest

The author declares no conflict of interest.

Author details

Sandro Misciagna
Neuroscience Department, Belcolle Hospital, Viterbo, Italy

*Address all correspondence to: sandromisciagna@yahoo.it

References

[1] Devinsky O, Gazzola D, LaFrance WC Jr. Differentiating between nonepileptic and epileptic seizures. Nature Reviews Neurology. 2011;7:210-220

[2] LaFrance JW, Schachter S. Historical Approaches to Treatments for Psychogenic Nonepileptic Seizures. New York: Cambridge University Press; 2010

[3] Liske E, Forster FM. Pseudoseizures: A problem in the diagnosis and management of epileptic patients. Neurology. 1964;**14**(1):41-49

[4] Asadi-Pooya AA, Brigo F, Mildon B, Nicholson TR. Terminology for psychogenic nonepileptic seizures: Making the case for "functional seizures". Epilepsy & Behavior. 2020;**104**:106895

[5] Kerr WT, Stern JM. We need a functioning name for PNES: Consider dissociative seizures. Epilepsy & Behavior. 2020;**105**:107002

[6] Brigo F, Igwe SC, Ausserer H, et al. Terminology of psychogenic nonepileptic seizures. Epilepsia. 2015;**56**(3):e21-e25

[7] Perez DL, Dworetzky BA, Dickerson BC, et al. An integrative neurocircuit perspective on psychogenic nonepileptic seizures and functional movement disorders: Neural functional unawareness. Clinical EEG and Neuroscience. 2015;**46**:4-15

[8] Benbadis SR, Allen HW. An estimate of the prevalence of psychogenic non-epileptic seizures. Seizure. 2000;**9**(4):280-281

[9] Asadi-Pooya AA, Sperling MR. Epidemiology of psychogenic nonepileptic seizures. Epilepsy & Behavior. 2015;**46**:60-65

[10] Salinsky M, Evrard C, Storzbach D, Pugh MJ. Psychiatric comorbidity in veterans with psychogenic seizures. Epilepsy & Behavior. 2012;**25**:345-349

[11] Hirtz D, Thurman DJ, Gwinn-Hardy K, Mohamed M, Chaudhuri AR, Zalutsky R. How common are the "common" neurologic disorders? Neurology. 2007;**68**:326-337

[12] Duncan R, Razvi S, Mulhern S. Newly presenting psychogenic nonepileptic seizures: Incidence, population characteristics, and early outcome from a prospective audit of a first seizure clinic. Epilepsy & Behavior. 2011;**20**:308-311

[13] Alsaadi TM, Marquez AV. Psychogenic nonepileptic seizures. American Family Physician. 2005;**72**(5):849-856

[14] Prerez DL, LaFrance WC. Nonepileptic seizures: An update review. CNS Spectrums. 2016;**21**(3):239-246

[15] Duncan R, Oto M. Predictors of antecedent factors in psychogenic nonepileptic attacks: Multivariate analysis. Neurology. 2008;**71**:1000-1005

[16] Reuber M. The etiology of psychogenic non-epileptic seizures: Toward a biopsychosocial model. Neurologic Clinics. 2009;**27**(4):909-924

[17] Dixit R, Popescu A, Bagic A, Ghearing G, Hendrickson R. Medical comorbidities in patients with psychogenic nonepileptic spells (PNES) referred for video-EEG monitoring. Epilepsy & Behavior. 2013;**28**:137-140

[18] Bodde NM, Brooks JL, Baker GA, Boon PA, Hendriksen JG, Aldenkamp AP.

Psychogenic non-epileptic seizures–diagnostic issues: A critical review. Clinical Neurology and Neurosurgery. Jan 2009;**111**(1):1-9. DOI: 10.1016/j.clineuro.2008.09.028. Epub 2008 Nov 18

[19] Gearhart MG, Brewerton TD. Psychogenic nonepileptic seizures associated with an eating disorder and PTSD are responsive to cognitive processing therapy. Case Rep Psychiatry. 2023;**2023**:5539951

[20] Direk N, Kulaksizoglu IB, Alpay K, Gurses C. Using personality disorders to distinguish between patients with psychogenic nonepileptic seizures and those with epileptic seizures. Epilepsy & Behavior. 2012;**23**:138-141

[21] Myers L, Perrine K, Lancman M, Fleming M, Lancman M. Psychological trauma in patients with psychogenic nonepileptic seizures: Trauma characteristics and those who develop PTSD. Epilepsy & Behavior. 2013;**28**:121-126

[22] Selkirk M, Duncan R, Oto M, Pelosi A. Clinical differences between patients with nonepileptic seizures who report antecedent sexual abuse and those who do not. Epilepsia. 2008;**49**:1446-1450

[23] Hingray C, Maillard L, Hubsch C, et al. Psychogenic nonepileptic seizures: Characterization of two distinct patient profiles on the basis of trauma history. Epilepsy & Behavior. 2011;**22**:532-536

[24] Chen DK, Izadyar S. Characteristics of psychogenic nonepileptic events among veterans with posttraumatic stress disorder: An association of semiology with the nature of trauma. Epilepsy & Behavior. 2010;**17**:188-192

[25] Asmussen SB, Kirlin KA, Gale SD, Chung SS. Differences in self-reported depressive symptoms between patients with epileptic and psychogenic nonepileptic seizures. Seizure: The Journal of the British Epilepsy Association. 2009;**18**:564-566

[26] Cohen ML, Testa SM, Pritchard JM, Zhu J, Hopp JL. Overlap between dissociation and other psychological characteristics in patients with psychogenic nonepileptic seizures. Epilepsy & Behavior. 2014;**34**:47-49

[27] Kaplan MJ, Dwivedi AK, Privitera MD, Isaacs K, Hughes C, Bowman M. Comparisons of childhood trauma, alexithymia, and defensive styles in patients with psychogenic non-epileptic seizures vs. epilepsy: Implications for the etiology of conversion disorder. Journal of Psychosomatic Research. 2013;**75**:142-146

[28] Brown RJ, Bouska JF, Frow A, et al. Emotional dysregulation, alexithymia, and attachment in psychogenic nonepileptic seizures. Epilepsy & Behavior. 2013;**29**:178-183

[29] Thompson AW, Hantke N, Phatak V, Chaytor N. The personality assessment inventory as a tool for diagnosing psychogenic nonepileptic seizures. Epilepsia. 2010;**51**:161-164

[30] Willment K, Hill M, Baslet G, Loring DW. Cognitive impairment and evaluation in psychogenic nonepileptic seizures: An integrated cognitive-emotional approach. Clinical EEG and Neuroscience. 2015;**46**:42-53

[31] Gale SD, Hill SW. Concurrent administration of the MMPI-2 and PAI in a sample of patients with epileptic or non-epileptic seizures: Implications for an inpatient epilepsy monitoring unit. Epilepsy & Behavior. 2012;**25**:181-184

[32] Prigatano GP, Kirlin KA. Self-appraisal and objective assessment of

cognitive and affective functioning in persons with epileptic and nonepileptic seizures. Epilepsy & Behavior. 2009;**14**:387-392

[33] O'Brien FM, Fortune GM, Dicker P, et al. Psychiatric and neuropsychological profiles of people with psychogenic nonepileptic seizures. Epilepsy & Behavior. 2015;**43**:39-45

[34] Gul A, Ahmad H. Cognitive deficits and emotion regulation strategies in patients with psychogenic nonepileptic seizures: A task-switching study. Epilepsy & Behavior. 2014;**32**:108-113

[35] Myers L, Zeng R, Perrine K, Lancman M, Lancman M. Cognitive differences between patients who have psychogenic nonepileptic seizures (PNESs) and posttraumatic stress disorder (PTSD) and patients who have PNESs without PTSD. Epilepsy & Behavior. 2014;**37**:82-86

[36] Asadi-Pooya AA. Psychogenic nonepileptic seizures: A concise review. Neurological Sciences. 2017;**38**(6):935-940

[37] Benbadis SR, Agrawal V, Tatum WO 4th. How many patients with psychogenic nonepileptic seizures also have epilepsy? Neurology. 2001;**57**(5):915-917

[38] Jafari A, Tavirani MS, Hamrach MP, et al. Psychogenic non-epileptic seizures; a narrative review. Archives of Academic Emergency Medicine. 2020;**8**(1):1-7

[39] Lobello K, Morgenlander J, Radtke R, Buschnell C. Video/EEG monitoring in the evaluation of paroxysmal behavioral events: Duration, effectiveness, and limitations. Epilepsy & Behavior. 2006;**8**(1):261-266

[40] Gröppel G, Kapitany T, Baumgartner C. Cluster analysis of clinical seizure semiology of psychogenic nonepileptic seizures. Epilepsia. 2000;**41**(5):610-614

[41] Lanzillotti AI, Sarudiansky M, Lombardi NR, et al. Updated review on the diagnosis and primary management of psychogenic nonepileptic seizure disorders. Neuropsychiatric Disease and Treatment. 2021;**17**:1825-1838

[42] Brigo F, Nardone R, Ausserer H, et al. The diagnostic value of urinary incontinence in the differential diagnosis of seizures. Seizure: The Journal of the British Epilepsy Association. 2013;**22**:85-90

[43] Saygi S, Katz A, Marks DA, Spencer SS. Frontal lobe partial seizures and psychogenic seizures: Comparison of clinical and ictal characteristics. Neurology. 1992;**42**(7):1274-1277

[44] Vossler DG, Haltiner AM, Schepp SK, et al. Ictal stuttering: A sign suggestive of psychogenic nonepileptic seizures. Neurology. 2004;**63**(3):516-519

[45] Burneo JG, Martin R, Powell T, et al. Teddy bears: An observational finding in patients with non-epileptic events. Neurology. 2003;**61**(5):714-715

[46] Goldstein LH, Mellers JD. Ictal symptoms of anxiety, avoidance behaviour, and dissociation in patients with dissociative seizures. Journal of Neurology, Neurosurgery, and Psychiatry. 2006;**77**(5):616-621

[47] Hendrickson R, Popescu A, Dixit R, et al. Panic attack symptoms differentiate patients with epilepsy from those with psychogenic nonepileptic spells (PNES). Epilepsy & Behavior. 2014;**37**:210-214

[48] American Psychiatric Association. Diagnostic and Statistical Manual

of Mental Disorders: DSM-IV-TR. Barcelona: Masson; 2002

[49] Avbersek A, Sisodiya S. Does the primary literature provide support for clinical signs used to distinguish psychogenic nonepileptic seizures from epileptic seizures? Journal of Neurology, Neurosurgery, and Psychiatry. 2010;**81**(7):719-725

[50] D'Alessio L, Giagante B, Oddo S, et al. Psychiatric disorders in patients with psychogenic non-epileptic seizures, with and without comorbid epilepsy. Seizure. 2006;**15**(5):333-339

[51] Devinsky O, Putman FW, Grafman J. Dissociation states and epilepsy. Neurology. 1989;**39**(6):835-840

[52] Schwabe M, Howell SJ, Reuber M. Differential diagnosis of seizure disorders: A conversation analytic approach. Social Science & Medicine. 2007;**65**(4):712-724

[53] Drazkowski JF, Chung SS. Differential diagnosis of epilepsy. Continuum (Minneap Minn). 2010;**16**(3 Epilepsy):36-56

[54] Syed TU, LaFrance WC Jr, Kahriman ES, et al. Can semiology predict psychogenic nonepileptic seizures? A prospective study. Annals of Neurology. 2011;**69**(6):997-1004

[55] Gasca-Salas C, Lang AE. Neurologic diagnostic criteria for functional neurologic disorders. Handbook of Clinical Neurology. 2016;**139**:193-212. DOI: 10.1016/B978-0-12-801772-2.00017-5. PMID: 27719839

[56] Alsaadi TM, Thieman C, Shatzel A, Farias S. Video-EEG telemetry can be a crucial tool for neurologists experienced in epilepsy when diagnosing seizure disorders. Seizure. 2004;**13**(1):32-34

[57] Ramani SV, Quesney LF, Olson D, et al. Diagnosis of hysterical seizures in epileptic patients. The American Journal of Psychiatry. 1980;**137**(6):705-709

[58] Parra J, Iriarte J, Kanner AM. Are we overusing the diagnosis of psychogenic non-epileptic events? Seizure. 1999;**8**(4):223-227

[59] Hoepner R, Labudda K, Schoendienst M, May TW, Bien CG, Brandt C. Informing patients about the impact of provocation methods increases the rate of psychogenic nonepileptic seizures during EEG recording. Epilepsy & Behavior. 2013;**28**:457-459

[60] Beniczky S, Conradsen I, Moldovan M, et al. Automated differentiation between epileptic and nonepileptic convulsive seizures. Annals of Neurology. 2015;**77**:348-351

[61] American Psychiatric Association. Diagnostic and Statistical Manual of Mental Disorders: DSM-5. VA: American Psychiatric Publishing; 2013

[62] World Health Organization. International Classification of Diseases and Related Health Problems, 10th Revision. Ginebra: WHO; 1992

[63] World Health Organization. International Classification of Diseases and Related Health Problems, 11th Revision. Ginebra: WHO; 2019

[64] Cianci V, Ferlazzo E, Condino F, et al. Rating scale for psychogenic nonepileptic seizures: Scale development and clinimetric testing. Epilepsy & Behavior. 2011;**21**(2):128-131

[65] Popkirov S, Gronheit W, Wellmer J. A systematic review of suggestive seizure induction for the diagnosis of psychogenic nonepileptic seizures. Seizure. 2015;**31**:124-132

[66] Petramfar P, Yaghoobi E, Nemati R, Asadi-Pooya AA. Serum

creatine phosphokinase is helpful in distinguishing generalized tonic–clonic seizures from psychogenic nonepileptic seizures and vasovagal syncope. Epilepsy & Behavior. 2009;**15**(3):330-332

[67] Willert C, Spitzer C, Kusserow S, Runge U. Serum neuron specific enolase, prolactin, and creatine kinase after epileptic and psychogenic non-epileptic seizures. Acta Neurologica Scandinavica. 2004;**109**(5):318-323

[68] Javali M, Acharya P, Shah S, Mahale R, Shetty P, Rangasetty S. Role of biomarkers in differentiating new-onset seizures from psychogenic nonepileptic seizures. Journal of Neurosciences in Rural Practice. 2017;**8**(04):581-584

[69] Sundararajan T, Tesar G, Jimenez X. Biomarkers in the diagnosis and study of psychogenic nonepileptic seizures: A systematic review. Seizure. 2016;**35**:11-22

[70] LaFrance WC Jr, Baker GA, Duncan R, Goldstein LH, Reuber M. Minimum requirements for the diagnosis of psychogenic nonepileptic seizures: A staged approach: A report from the international league against epilepsy nonepileptic seizures task force. Epilepsia. 2013a;**54**(11):2005-2018

[71] LaFrance WC Jr, Reuber M, Goldstein LH. Management of psychogenic nonepileptic seizures. Epilepsia. 2013b;**54**(Suppl. 1):53-67

[72] LaFrance WC Jr, Deluca M, Machan JT, Fava JL. Traumatic brain injury and psychogenic nonepileptic seizures yield worse outcomes. Epilepsia. 2013c;**54**:718-725

[73] Zhang S-W, Liu Y-X. Changes of serum adrenocorticotropic hormone and cortisol levels during sleep seizures. Neuroscience Bulletin. 2008;**24**(2):84-88

[74] Bakvis P, Spinhoven P, Giltay EJ, et al. Basal hypercortisolism and trauma in patients with psychogenic nonepileptic seizures. Epilepsia. 2010;**51**:752-759

[75] Bakvis P, Spinhoven P, Roelofs K. Basal cortisol is positively correlated to threat vigilance in patients with psychogenic nonepileptic seizures. Epilepsy & Behavior. 2009;**16**:558-560

[76] Winterdahl M, Miani A, Vercoe MJ, Ciovica A, Uber-Zak L, Rask CU, et al. Vulnerability to psychogenic nonepileptic seizures is linked to low neuropeptide Y levels. Stress. 2017;**20**(6):589-597

[77] Guilliams TG, Edwards L. Chronic stress and the HPA axis. The Standard. 2010;**9**(2):1-12

[78] Heim C, Young LJ, Newport DJ, Mletzko T, Miller AH, Nemeroff CB. Lower CSF oxytocin concentrations in women with a history of childhood abuse. Molecular Psychiatry. 2009;**14**(10):954-958

[79] Hertting A, Theorell T. Physiological changes associated with downsizing of personnel and reorganisation in the health care sector. Psychotherapy and Psychosomatics. 2002;**71**(2):117-122

[80] Green M, Matheson S, Shepherd A, Weickert C, Carr V. Brain-derived neurotrophic factor levels in schizophrenia: A systematic review with meta-analysis. Molecular Psychiatry. 2011;**16**(9):960-972

[81] Aydin S, Dag E, Ozkan Y, Arslan O, Koc G, Bek S, et al. Time-dependent changes in the serum levels of prolactin, nesfatin-1 and ghrelin as a marker of epileptic attacks young male patients. Peptides. 2011;**32**(6):1276-1280

[82] Numakawa T, Suzuki S, Kumamaru E, Adachi N, Richards M, Kunugi H. BDNF function and intracellular signalling in neurons.

Histology and Histopathology. 2010 Feb;**25**(2):237-258

[83] LaFrance WC Jr, Leaver K, Stopa EG, Papandonatos GD, Blum AS. Decreased serum BDNF levels in patients with epileptic and psychogenic nonepileptic seizures. Neurology. 2010a;**75**:1285-1291

[84] Deveci A, Aydemir O, Taskin O, Taneli F, Esen-Danaci A. Serum brain-derived neurotrophic factor levels in conversion disorder: Comparative study with depression. Psychiatry and Clinical Neurosciences. 2007;**61**(5):571-573

[85] Morales-Medina JC, Dumont Y, Quirion R. A possible role of neuropeptide Y in depression and stress. Brain Research. 2010;**1314**:194-205

[86] Nishikimi T, Kuwahara K, Nakao K. Current biochemistry, molecular biology, and clinical relevance of natriuretic peptides. Journal of Cardiology. 2011;**57**(2):131-140

[87] Ceylan M, Yalcin A, Bayraktutan OF, Laloglu E. Serum NT-pro CNP levels in epileptic seizure, psychogenic nonepileptic seizure, and healthy subjects. Neurological Sciences. 2018;**39**(12):2135-2139

[88] Arthuis M, Micoulaud-Franchi JA, Bartolomei F, McGonigal A, Guedj E. Resting cortical PET metabolic changes in psychogenic non-epileptic seizures (PNES). Journal of Neurology, Neurosurgery, and Psychiatry. 2015;**86**(10):1106-1112

[89] van der Kruijs SJ, Bodde NM, Vaessen MJ, et al. Functional connectivity of dissociation in patients with psychogenic non-epileptic seizures. Journal of Neurology, Neurosurgery, and Psychiatry. 2012;**83**:239-247

[90] Ding J, An D, Liao W, et al. Abnormal functional connectivity density in psychogenic non-epileptic seizures. Epilepsy Research. 2014;**108**:1184-1194

[91] van der Kruijs SJ, Jagannathan SR, Bodde NM, et al. Resting-state networks and dissociation in psychogenic non-epileptic seizures. Journal of Psychiatric Research. 2014;**54**:126-133

[92] Li R, Liu K, Ma X, et al. Altered functional connectivity patterns of the insular subregions in psychogenic nonepileptic seizures. Brain Topography. 2015a;**28**:636-645

[93] Li R, Li Y, An D, Gong Q, Zhou D, Chen H. Altered regional activity and inter-regional functional connectivity in psychogenic non-epileptic seizures. Scientific Reports. 2015b;**5**:11635

[94] Labate A, Cerasa A, Mula M, et al. Neuroanatomic correlates of psychogenic nonepileptic seizures: A cortical thickness and VBM study. Epilepsia. 2011;**53**:377-385

[95] Ristic AJ, Dakovic M, Kerr M, Kovacevic M, Parojcic A, Sokic D. Cortical thickness, surface area and folding in patients with psychogenic nonepileptic seizures. Epilepsy Research. 2015;**112**:84-91

[96] Hernando KA, Szaflarski JP, Ver Hoef LW, Lee S, Allendorfer JB. Uncinate fasciculus connectivity in patients with psychogenic nonepileptic seizures: A preliminary diffusion tensor tractography study. Epilepsy & Behavior. 2015;**45**:68-73

[97] Barzegaran E, Carmeli C, Rossetti AO, Frackowiak RS, Knyazeva MG. Weakened functional connectivity in patients with psychogenic non-epileptic seizures (PNES) converges on basal ganglia. Journal of Neurology, Neurosurgery, and Psychiatry. 2016;**87**(3):332-337

[98] Ponnusamy A, Marques JL, Reuber M. Comparison of heart rate variability parameters during complex partial seizures and psychogenic nonepileptic seizures. Epilepsia. 2012;**53**:1314-1321

[99] Reinsberger C, Perez DL, Murphy MM, Dworetzky BA. Pre- and postictal, not ictal, heart rate distinguishes complex partial and psychogenic nonepileptic seizures. Epilepsy & Behavior. 2012;**23**:68-70

[100] Martin RC, Gilliam FG, Kilgore M, Faught E, Kuzniecky R. Improved health care resource utilization following video-EEG- confirmed diagnosis of nonepileptic psychogenic seizures. Seizure. 1998;**7**(5):385-390

[101] Duncan R, Horwood J, Razvi S, Mulhern S. Psychogenic nonepileptic seizures that remit when the diagnosis is given: Just good luck? Epilepsy & Behavior. 2020;**102**:106667

[102] Thompson R, Isaac CL, Rowse G, Tooth CL, Reuber M. What is it like to receive a diagnosis of nonepileptic seizures? Epilepsy & Behavior. 2009;**14**(3):508-515

[103] Baslet G, Roiko A, Prensky E. Heterogeneity in psychogenic nonepileptic seizures: Understanding the role of psychiatric and neurological factors. Epilepsy & Behavior. 2010;**17**(2):236-241

[104] Beck AT. The current state of cognitive therapy. Archives of General Psychiatry. 2005;**62**(9):953-959

[105] Goldstein LH, Chalder T, Chigwedere C, et al. Cognitive–behavioral therapy for psychogenic nonepileptic seizures: A pilot RCT. Neurology. 2010;**74**(24):1986-1994

[106] Howlett S, Reuber M. An augmented model of brief psychodynamic interpersonal therapy for patients with nonepileptic seizures. Psychotherapy. 2009;**46**(1):125-138

[107] Baslet G, Ehlert A, Oser M, Dworetzky BA. Mindfulness-based therapy for psychogenic nonepileptic seizures. Epilepsy & Behavior. 2020;**103**:106534

[108] Hayes SC, Luoma JB, Bond FW, Masuda A, Lillis J. Acceptance and commitment therapy: Model, processes and outcomes. Behaviour Research and Therapy. 2006;**44**:1-25

[109] Gaudiano BA. The "Third Wave" behavior therapies in context: Review of Hayes et al.'s (2004)Mindfulness and acceptance: Expanding the cognitive-behavioral tradition and Hayes and Strosahl's (2004) a practical guide to acceptance and commitment therapy. Cognitive and Behavioral Practice. 2006;**13**(1):101-104. DOI:10.1016/j.cbpra.2006.01.002

[110] Barrett-Naylor R, Gresswell DM, Dawson DL. The effectiveness and acceptability of a guided self-help acceptance and commitment therapy (ACT) intervention for psychogenic nonepileptic seizures. Epilepsy & Behavior. 2018;**88**:332-340

[111] Zaroff CM, Myers L, Barr WB, Luciano D, Devinsky O. Group psychoeducation as treatment for psychological nonepileptic seizures. Epilepsy & Behavior. 2004;**5**(4):587-592

[112] Chen DK, Maheshwari A, Franks R, Trolley GC, Robinson JS, Hrachovy RA. Brief group psychoeducation for psychogenic nonepileptic seizures: A neurologist-initiated program in an epilepsy center. Epilepsia. 2014;**55**:156-166

[113] Mayor R, Brown RJ, Cock H, et al. A feasibility study of a brief psycho-educational intervention for psychogenic

nonepileptic seizures. Seizure. 2013;**22**(9):760-765

[114] Krawetz P, Fleisher W, Pillay N, Staley D, Arnett J, Maher J. Family functioning in subjects with pseudoseizures and epilepsy. The Journal of Nervous and Mental Disease. 2001;**189**(1):38-43

[115] Metin SZ, Ozmen M, Metin B, Talasman S, Yeni SN, Ozkara C. Treatment with group psychotherapy for chronic psychogenic nonepileptic seizures. Epilepsy & Behavior. 2013;**28**(1):91-94

[116] de Oliveira SN, Benute GR, Santiago A, Marchiori PE, Lucia MC. Psychogenic non-epileptic seizures and psychoanalytical treatment: Results. Revista da Associação Médica Brasileira. 2014;**60**(6):577-584

[117] Foa EB, Hembree E, Rothbaum B. Prolonged Exposure Therapy for PTSD: Emotional Processing of Traumatic Experiences, Therapist Guide. 2 edn. Treatments That Work. New York: Oxford Academic; 1 Aug 2019. DOI: 10.1093/med-psych/9780190926939.001.0001 [Accessed: May 7, 2024]

[118] Myers L, Vaidya-Mathur U, Lancman M. Prolonged exposure therapy for the treatment of patients diagnosed with psychogenic non-epileptic seizures (PNES) and post-traumatic stress disorder (PTSD). Epilepsy & Behavior. 2017;**66**:86-92

[119] Demirci OO, Sagaltici E. Eye movement desensitization and reprocessing treatment in functional neurological symptom disorder with psychogenic nonepileptic seizures: A study of two cases. Clinical Child Psychology and Psychiatry. 2021;**26**(4):1196-1207

[120] LaFrance WC Jr, Keitner GI, Papandonatos GD, et al. Pilot pharmacologic randomized controlled trial for psychogenic nonepileptic seizures. Neurology. 2010b;**75**:1166-1173

[121] LaFrance WC Jr, Baird GL, Barry JJ, et al. Multicenter pilot treatment trial for psychogenic nonepileptic seizures: A randomized clinical trial. JAMA Psychiatry. 2014;**71**:997-1005

[122] LaFrance WC Jr, Wincze J. Treating Nonepieptic Seizures: Therapist Guide. New York: Oxford Univeristy Press; 2015

[123] Baslet G, Dworetzky B, Perez DL, Oser M. Treatment of psychogenic nonepileptic seizures: Updated review and findings from a mindfulness-based intervention case series. Clinical EEG and Neuroscience. 2015;**46**:54-64

[124] Duncan R, Graham CD, Oto M. Neurologist assessment of reactions to the diagnosis of psychogenic nonepileptic seizures: Relationship to short- and long-term outcomes. Epilepsy & Behavior. 2014;**41**:79-82

[125] McKenzie P, Oto M, Russell A, Pelosi A, Duncan R. Early outcomes and predictors in 260 patients with psychogenic nonepileptic attacks. Neurology. 2010;**74**:64-69

Chapter 4

Navigating the Shadows: Understanding and Managing Persistent Somatic Symptoms in Cancer Survivors

Val Bellman

Abstract

The purpose of this chapter is to provide healthcare professionals, researchers and caregivers with insights on persistent somatic symptoms afflicting cancer survivors. These symptoms, including pain, fatigue, gastrointestinal distress, sexual dysfunction, respiratory issues, and cardiovascular, neurological and musculoskeletal complications often endure long after treatment completion, negatively impacting quality of life. Certain populations like childhood cancer survivors and those receiving intensive chemotherapy have higher somatic symptom burden. Possible mechanisms include accelerated aging, somatization tendencies, treatment side effects, mood disorders, and comorbidities. Assessing patient-reported outcomes and screening tools can facilitate early detection and management. Treatment strategies encompass pharmacological and nonpharmacological modalities targeting specific symptoms. Overall somatic symptom burden correlates with psychological distress and disability among survivors. Tailored, patient-centric rehabilitation programs over the cancer trajectory, from pretreatment through long-term survivorship, can mitigate symptoms. More research on persistent somatic complications is warranted to optimize evidence-based care for survivors' multifaceted needs.

Keywords: cancer survivors, somatic symptoms, persistent pain, fatigue, psychological distress, quality of life, rehabilitation

1. Introduction

Imagine a cancer survivor, who, after undergoing rigorous treatments and conquering the disease, finds themself grappling with unexplained physical symptoms that persist long after their remission. Despite their triumph over cancer, they feel trapped in the shadows of persistent somatic symptoms, impacting their daily life. Unfortunately, this experience is not unique, as many cancer survivors face similar challenges even after their battle with the disease has ended. In this chapter, we delve into the often-overlooked aspect of persistent somatic symptoms in individuals who have emerged victorious against cancer. Survivors often face a range of physical, psychological, and emotional challenges that can persist long after treatment ends. These symptoms, which can manifest in various forms and intensities, significantly impact survivors' daily functioning and overall quality of life.

By shedding light on this topic, we aim to provide healthcare professionals, researchers, and caregivers with valuable insights and evidence-based approaches to alleviate suffering and improve the lives of cancer survivors.

To ensure the depth and accuracy of our findings, we conducted a meticulous review of the existing literature on persistent somatic symptoms in cancer survivors. By examining a wide array of studies, we aim to present a comprehensive synthesis of current knowledge and identify gaps that warrant further investigation.

2. Prevalence and impact of persistent somatic symptoms in cancer survivors

Persistent somatic symptoms can substantially impact cancer survivors' quality of life and well-being. These symptoms encompass physical and psychological issues like pain, fatigue, anxiety, depression, and sleep problems [1–3]. Long-term rare cancer survivors commonly report tiredness/lack of energy as the most prevalent and bothersome symptom [3]. Emotional distress symptoms like depression, anxiety, and somatization are common in childhood cancer survivors [4]. Notably, symptoms can persist long-term after treatment as late effects of cancer or therapy [5]. Comorbidities strongly predict early mortality in survivors [6]. Studies consistently link somatic symptom severity and frequency to fear of recurrence in childhood cancer survivors [7]. Symptom burden profoundly impacts health-related quality of life; survivors with high physical, somatic and psychological symptoms report remarkably poor physical and mental quality of life [8]. Somatic symptoms are associated with disability and increased healthcare use in cancer patients with pain/depression [9].

The prevalence and persistence of these symptoms can vary based on factors such as age, comorbidity, race, and cancer type. For instance, older breast cancer survivors commonly report symptoms such as cardiotoxic effects, peripheral neuropathy, cognitive problems, fatigue, anxiety, depression, and sleep disturbances [1]. Similarly, racial and ethnic disparities have been observed in the physical and mental health outcomes of cancer survivors, with Black, Hispanic, and Indigenous survivors experiencing poorer health outcomes [10]. Moreover, sexual orientation and racial/ethnic differences have been found to influence the physical and mental health outcomes of female and male cancer survivors [11]. For example, prostate cancer survivors with high symptom burden require more supportive information and tailored long-term survivorship care to address their needs effectively [12].

2.1 Factors contributing to higher risk of persistent somatic symptoms in certain survivor populations

Research suggests childhood cancer survivors may experience premature aging, potentially due to cancer therapy exposure leading to cellular senescence, reduced telomere length, epigenetic changes, somatic mutations, and mitochondrial DNA issues [13]. Biological pathways likely explain the occurrence of psychosomatic symptoms like pain, fatigue, and weakness in conditions such as somatization, depression, and chronic fatigue [14]. In cancer, somatization manifests as somatic symptoms including pain,

Factor	Description	Reference
High Prevalence	The manifestation of psychological distress through physical symptoms is a significant concern among 50% of cancer survivors.	[23]
Type of cancer	Survivors of childhood cancer may experience higher levels of depression, anxiety, and somatization	[24]
Psychosocial Factors	Immigrants have elevated levels of somatization and anxiety Higher rates of depression and relationship difficulty in LGBTQ community	[17, 25]
Demographic Factors	Somatization is associated with higher age, male sex, low education, and living alone.	[26, 27]

Table 1.
Somatization in cancer survivors.

fatigue, appetite changes, and low energy [15]. Minor bodily symptoms may be cognitively linked to fear of recurrence, influencing survivors' well-being [16].

All survivors have poorer psychological health than cancer-free individuals, emphasizing the psychological impact of survivorship [17]. Childhood leukemia, Hodgkin's disease, and lymphoma survivors who had intensive chemotherapy have an increased risk of depression and somatic distress [18]. Factors like female sex, low education, income, and unemployment are associated with increased physical distress in childhood cancer survivors [19]. Psychological distress persists in 20–40% of survivors, highlighting its enduring impact [20]. Long-term psychoactive drug use is associated with more somatic symptoms in psychiatric patients [21]. Worsening physical health, pain, and ending analgesics predict persistent distress in survivors [22]. **Table 1** summarizes somatization aspects in survivors.

3. Characteristics of persistent somatic symptoms in cancer survivors

Somatic symptoms are prevalent among cancer survivors. These symptoms include pain, fatigue, anxiety, depression, and somatic distress. Cunningham et al. highlighted that somatic symptoms, such as pain and fatigue, are common after childhood cancer and are associated with greater fear of cancer recurrence and poorer health-related quality of life [7]. Moreover, Heathcote et al. emphasized the prevalence and burden of somatic symptoms, particularly pain and fatigue, in adult survivors of childhood cancer [28]. Tuman et al. also found that breast cancer survivors with a tendency to make threatening interpretations experienced overall problematic somatic symptoms [29]. Furthermore, fear of cancer recurrence has been linked to somatic symptoms and perceived stress among cancer survivors [30].

3.1 Chronic pain in cancer survivors

Chronic pain is a common issue among cancer survivors, significantly impacting their daily functioning [31]. Studies have shown that chronic pain is prevalent and disabling, affecting a substantial proportion of cancer survivors [32]. Pain is one of the most distressing symptoms experienced by cancer survivors, with a notable impact on their quality of life [33]. However, there is a lack of recognition among clinicians regarding the frequency of chronic pain in this population, which may lead to underestimation of its prevalence and severity [34, 35]. Therefore, tailored policies, guidelines, and comprehensive training for healthcare professionals in pain management are necessary to address the complexity of chronic pain in cancer survivors [36]. The management of pain in cancer survivors presents various challenges, including social and demographic inequalities in barriers to cancer pain management [37]. The use of opioids in cancer survivors with chronic pain raises concerns, and advanced therapeutic strategies may be necessary to ensure prolonged pain control [38]. **Figure 1** summarizes the most common indications for opiates in this population.

Additionally, cancer-specific psychosocial factors, such as pain catastrophizing and multisite pain, contribute to the pain experience in cancer survivors [39]. Healthcare professionals must manage the needs of cancer survivors in a manner that acknowledges the burden of pain in the context of other symptoms and morbidities experienced by long-term survivors [40]. Various interventions have been explored to address chronic pain in cancer survivors, including acupuncture, cognitive behavioral therapy, and breathing exercises, with some evidence of positive effects for pain relief [41, 42]. Moreover, the evaluation of medications and self-management techniques for controlling neuropathic symptoms in cancer survivors highlights the multifaceted approach required to address the complexities of pain management in this population [43]. **Figure 2** summarizes pharmacological pain management in this population.

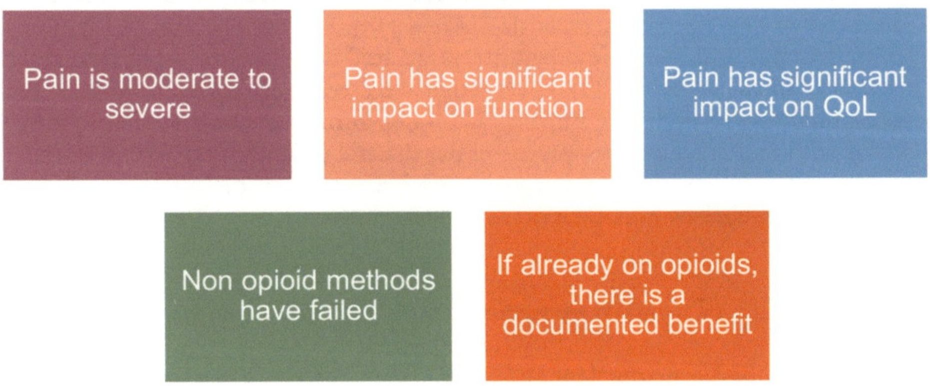

Figure 1.
Indications for opioids in cancer survivors.

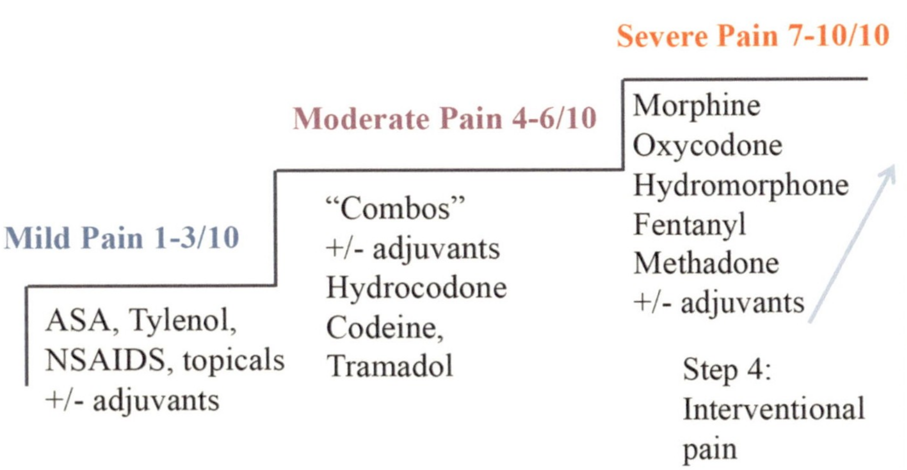

Figure 2.
World Health Organization (WHO) step ladder approach.

3.2 Chronic fatigue in cancer survivors

The prevalence of moderate to severe fatigue among cancer survivors has been reported to be as high as 66.1%, with a significant impact on their quality of life [44]. Studies have shown that fatigue is prevalent not only in breast cancer survivors but also in survivors of lung, colorectal, prostate, and other types of cancer [45]. **Table 2** summarizes various instruments to screen or measure fatigue.

Furthermore, fatigue has been found to co-occur with other symptoms such as depression, insomnia, neuropathy, and pain, contributing to the overall burden experienced by cancer survivors [46]. It has also been noted that fatigue may persist for months after the completion of cancer treatment, affecting 30–60% of cancer

Screening Tool	Description
Brief Screening Tools	• VAS 0–10 scales • Multi-symptom screening scales: ESAS, MSAS
Unidimensional Scales (physical impact of CRF)	• Functional Assessment of Cancer Therapy Fatigue (FACT-F) • Brief Fatigue Inventory (BFI) • EORTC QLQ C30
Multidimensional Scales (physical, cognitive, affective)	• Fatigue Symptom Inventory (FSI) • Revised Piper Fatigue Scale • Chalder Fatigue Scale / Fatigue Questionnaire
ICD-10 Diagnostic Criteria Guided Clinical Diagnosis	Diagnosis if six or more of the following symptoms are present daily or nearly daily during same 2 weeks in past month and at least one of symptoms is significant fatigue: • fatigue (diminished energy, increased need to rest disproportionate to • change in activity) • generalized weakness, limb heaviness • diminished concentration, attention • decreased motivation, interest in activities • insomnia, hypersomnia • non-restorative sleep • struggle to overcome inactivity • emotional reactivity to feeling fatigued (sadness, frustration, irritability) • difficulty with daily tasks because of fatigue • short-term memory problems • post-exertional malaise lasting several hours • Symptoms cause clinically significant distress or • impairment in social, occupational, or other important • areas of functioning • Evidence from history, physical examination, or • laboratory findings that symptoms are consequence of • cancer or cancer therapy • Symptoms not primarily consequence of comorbid • psychiatric disorders such as major depression, • somatization or somatoform disorder, or delirium

ESAS: The Edmonton Symptom Assessment System.
VAS: Visual Analogue Scale.
MSAS: The Memorial Symptom Assessment Scale.
EORTC QLQ-C30: The EORTC Core Quality of Life questionnaire.

Table 2.
Screening for chronic fatigue syndrome.

Psychogenic	Organic disease
Mostly <6 months and fluctuates in severity	6 months
Related to various stressors	Obvious psychosocial sctressors are often absent
Sleeping disturbance with either insomnia or eary morning awakening	Varies. May be present but often related to the underlying illness
Worse in the morning, may be alleviated by activity	Less in the morning and worsened with activity
Multiple and nonspecific complaints along with a normal exam	Fewer and more specific symptoms. Exam may suggest potential underlying problem

Table 3.
Ethnology of cancer fatigue.

Chronic fatigue in cancer survivors	Depression in cancer survivors
Fatigue much more common than depression (60–90% vs. 20–25%)	Depression more likely in presence of • hopelessness, worthlessness, guilt • history or family history of depression
Depressive symptoms due to fatigue are often less severe and are attributed to consequences of fatigue by patients	Suicidal ideations, desire for death are not common in patients with fatigue

Table 4.
Fatigue and depression in cancer survivors.

survivors [47]. **Table 3** summarizes possible underlying mechanisms behind chronic fatigue in cancer survivors.

Furthermore, chronic fatigue has been found to be strongly associated with depression in cancer survivors, indicating a potential interplay between these two conditions [48]. While both fatigue and depression are prevalent among cancer survivors, it is essential to differentiate between these two conditions. **Table 4** summarizes core findings and differences.

The management of fatigue in cancer survivors is a complex challenge, as there is currently no somatic strategy specifically tailored to address this issue [49]. Furthermore, the experience of chronic fatigue post-treatment can have a profound impact on the family and social dynamics of cancer survivors [50]. **Table 5** summarizes the main treatment strategies.

Interventions for Fatigue	Description
Depression treatment	1. Typical antidepressants • selective serotonin reuptake inhibitors (SSRIs) may be better tolerated than others • bupropion may be more activating (similar in structure to stimulants) • novel agents (venlafaxine, nefazodone, mirtazapine) 2. Psychostimulants • methylphenidate, dextroamphetamine, modafinil, amodafinil
Nonpharmacologic interventions	• Physical Activity / Aerobic Exercise [51] • Energy conservation and restoration • Sleep restoration, UV Light Therapy

Interventions for Fatigue	Description
	Psychotherapies: • Cognitive Behavioral Therapy • Mindfulness Based Stress Reduction • Psycho-educational, Supportive Counseling, journal [52, 53]. • Meditation/Relaxation/Yoga • Acupuncture, Quigong • Nutritional Counseling/Supplements
Pharmacologic interventions	1. Psychostimulants • methylphenidate (2.5 to 30 mg once or twice daily or higher) • dextroamphetamine (2.5 to 30 mg once or twice daily or higher) • modafinil (100 to 400 mg/day) • amodafinil (150–250 mg/day) 2. Corticosteroids • dexamethasone (1 to 3 mg bid) • prednisone (5 to 10 mg bid): limited data; at least transient symptom improvement; long-term benefit not demonstrated 3. Pharmacologic interventions with L-carnitine • Patients with advanced cancer are at risk for carnitine deficiency because of low intake and increased renal loss. 4. Anticytokine agents (thalidomide, pentoxifylline, cox-2 inhibitors) 5. Other agents (donepezil, megestrol acetate, amantadine, anabolic steroids, antidepressants, sleep aids) 6. Supplements: ginseng, Vit D, others

Table 5.
Management of chronic fatigue.

3.3 Impact of cognitive impairment on somatic symptoms in cancer survivors

Research has shown that long-term survivors are at risk for neurocognitive impairment due to multiple sources of risk [54]. The lack of information regarding cognitive impairment has been found to negatively impact the work and work capacity of cancer survivors [55]. Chemotherapy has been implicated in cognitive abnormalities in cancer survivors, including impairments of memory, attention, processing speed, and executive function [56]. Moreover, aging cancer survivors may report new-onset neurocognitive impairments, and there is a need to identify risk factors associated with such impairments [57]. **Table 6** outlines assessment and diagnosis of cognitive impairment in cancer survivors.

History	• Time course of cognitive decline (correlation with cancer, chemo, hospitalization) • Fluctuations/Sleep wake cycle • Assess for pain and discomfort • Cognitive, functional, behavioral history (current and baseline) with collateral from family and caregivers • h/o delirium or dementia, seizures, falls, h/o ICU stay • Medication list/ chemotherapy or other cancer therapies • ETOH, benzodiazepines • Vascular risk factors • Family history of neurodegenerative disorders
Examination	1. Mental Status Examination and cognitive/neuropsychological testing 2. Physical examination 3. Neurological examination (frontal release signs, gait, asterixis, EPS, focal findings)

Diagnostic Work Up	• Basic Metabolic Panel: Na, K, Ca, Mg/ BUN and • creatinine/ LFTs/ Albumin • CBC (WBC, Hemoglobin/Hematocrit, MCV, Platelets) • Thyroid function tests, RPR, FTA-ABS, Vitamin B12 • Thiamine • EKG • UA/Cultures • ABG/CXR • Ammonia • EEG/ Brain Imaging/LP
Differential Diagnosis	• Delirium, • Depression, Anxiety, Adjustment disorders • Fatigue, Sleep Disorders (insomnia, sleep apnea), • Substance Use Disorders, • Paraneoplastic syndromes, • • Mild or Major Neurocognitive Disorder

Table 6.
Assessment of cognitive impairment in cancer survivors.

Cognitive rehabilitation has been proposed as a potential intervention, as concerns about impaired cognition are one of the most frequently reported post-treatment symptoms in cancer survivors [58]. Physical activity has been associated with better neurocognitive function in cancer survivors, suggesting a potential avenue for intervention [59]. The National Comprehensive Cancer Network recommends pharmacologic interventions as a last line of therapy:

- Psychostimulants: methylphenidate, dextroamphetamine
- Wakefulness-promoting agents: modafinil, armodafinil
- Cholinesterase inhibitors: Donepezil, rivastigmine
- NMDA-antagonists: Memantine
- Bupropion, atomoxetine

Table 7 summarizes neuromodulation strategies utilized in cancer survivors.

Strategy	**Description**
Neurofeedback	Promising results in breast cancer patients.
Repetitive transcranial magnetic stimulation	Currently, no studies in cancer patients.
Transcranial Direct Current Stimulation	• Non-invasive brain stimulation technology • Studied in patients with depression, pain syndromes, stroke, Alzheimer's, and Parkinson's disease in non-cancer settings with promising clinical evidence.

Table 7.
Neuromodulation strategies for cognitive difficulties in survivorship.

3.4 Impact of sleep disorders on somatic symptoms in survivors

Sleep disorders and somatic symptoms are prevalent among cancer survivors, impacting their quality of life and psychological well-being. Statistically, sleep medication use is prevalent among cancer survivors, with the prevalence of insomnia symptoms being nearly 40% in this population [60]. Research indicates that adult survivors of childhood cancer are more likely to experience fatigue, sleep disturbance, and daytime sleepiness [61]. For instance, a study by Schlarb et al. found that self-reported sleep quality, sleep onset latency, sleep disturbances, use of sleep medications, and daytime dysfunctioning were significant predictors of somatoform syndrome, while sleep efficiency and sleep duration indirectly influenced somatic complaints [62]. Insomnia severity is directly related to habitual somatic complaints and pain intensity [63]. Similarly, Sun et al. indicated that a high level of somatic symptoms exacerbates the adverse effects on sleep disturbance, emphasizing the bidirectional nature of the relationship [64]. **Table 8** summarizes general principles and interventions in cancer patients and survivors with sleep problems.

3.5 Sexual dysfunction in cancer survivors

Research shows sexual dysfunction is a prevalent issue among cancer survivors, especially childhood and young adult survivors. A review highlighted adolescent and young adult survivors experience substantial sexual dysfunction [65]. Another review identified the prevalence and risk factors for sexual dysfunction in childhood cancer survivors, emphasizing its link to quality of life and psychosocial outcomes [18]. Studies show childhood cancer survivors may experience sexual difficulties and delays in milestones due to the cancer's impact on psychosexual development [66]. Sexual dysfunction is prevalent among female childhood cancer survivors, significantly impacting their psychosexual functioning [67]. There is an increased risk of sexual dysfunction in young adult survivors of childhood cancer, indicating a need for support in this population [68]. Another study emphasized the lack of information on sexual health for male childhood cancer survivors, showing further research and support is needed [69]. Standardized nursing care interventions reduced sexual dysfunction in cervical cancer survivors, underscoring potential benefits of targeted

Intervention	Characteristics
Nonpharmacological Interventions	• Cognitive-behavioral therapy for insomnia (CBT-I) (+) strong evidence in cancer patients with therapeutic effects maintained long term. • Exercise Interventions: regular aerobic exercises, even of different durations and • weekly volumes, benefits patient sleep quality.
Pharmacological Interventions	• The American Academy of Sleep Medicine does not recommend sleep medications for longer than 4 weeks. • The NCCN Survivorship Guidelines recommends assessment every 1 to 3 months to determine ongoing need for medications. • All medications have been shown to be more effective than placebo at improving short-term sleep outcomes in the general population. • The potential benefits of pharmacologic therapy on sleep quality and daytime function are balanced against the risk of side effects and dependence with long-term use.

Table 8.
Management of sleep difficulties in cancer survivors.

ASK	About sexual function at regular intervals
ASSESS	Using the Brief Sexual Symptom Checklist as a primary screening tool
REVIEW	Present and past sexual history and sexual concerns
DISCUSS	How cancer treatment has affected sexual functioning, intimacy, treatment-associated infertility and, if indicated, provide appropriate referrals
DIRECT	Patients to needed resources

Table 9.
Guidelines of sexual dysfunction.

interventions [70]. These findings demonstrate sexual dysfunction is a common issue among survivors that interventions may help address. **Table 9** summarizes NCCN guidelines regarding sexual dysfunction.

3.6 Weight loss in cancer survivors

Weight loss and poor appetite are significant concerns among cancer patients and survivors. Another study highlighted that intermittent claudication and appetite loss are common among breast cancer survivors and are associated with cardiac dysfunction and mood disorders [71]. Similarly, it was found that self-reported distress among older cancer survivors was associated with weight change and poor appetite [72]. Additionally, identified appetite changes as one of the indicators of physical wellbeing in cancer survivors, emphasizing its impact on quality of life [73]. **Table 10** summarizes the differences between starvation and cancer/post-treatment weight loss.

Furthermore, emphasized the consequences of weight loss for cancer survivors as a crucial issue in survivorship research, highlighting the need for interventions to address this concern [74]. Other authors also identified appetite loss as a part of a cluster of symptoms in breast cancer survivors, indicating its impact on their quality of life [75]. Research highlighted the importance of maintaining a healthy weight for cancer survivors, emphasizing the potential benefits for their overall well-being [76]. In addition, weight loss interventions have been studied in the context of cancer survivorship. Reported that behaviorally based weight loss interventions for breast cancer survivors resulted in significant weight losses, indicating the potential effectiveness of such interventions. **Table 11** summarizes pharmacological and nonpharmacological management of cancer and post-treatment weight loss in cancer survivors.

Starvation	Cancer/Post-Treatment Weight Loss
Loss of adipose tissue	Loss of fat and lean muscles
Hunger is present, significant	No hunger, no concerns about food
Decreased resting energy	Increased resting energy expenditure
No specific mediators or markers	Pro-inflammatory cytokines

Table 10.
Weight and appetite loss and cancer cachexia.

Strategy	Description
Counseling	The nutritional counseling: liberalizing diet restrictions, encouraging patients to eat frequent small meals with preferably the bulk of calorie intake occurring in the morning.
Nonpharmacological Management	• Ensuring sufficient energy and protein intake (nutritional support, consultation with a nutritionist) • Maintaining body weight, physical activity and muscle mass (exercise, PT)
Pharmacological Management	1. Appetite Stimulants • corticosteroids, cannabinoids, progesterone analogs, and serotonin modulators (olanzapine, mirtazapine). 2. Anabolic Agents • anabolic steroids • Growth hormone, ghrelin analogs 3. Cytokine and metabolic inhibitors • Eicosapentaenoic acid • Thalidomide

Table 11.
Weight and appetite loss management.

3.7 Gastrointestinal distress in cancer survivors

Nausea and vomiting are very common in cancer patients, including survivors. Research shows 70–80% of chemotherapy patients experience these symptoms [77], which continue into survivorship and hurt quality of life [78]. Over 60% of terminally ill patients have nausea and vomiting in their last 6 weeks [79]. Managing these symptoms is crucial for survivors' wellbeing. Studies suggest high protein intake can lessen nausea and vomiting [80]. Acupressure has been explored to treat chemotherapy-induced nausea and vomiting [81]. Aromatherapy with ginger may alleviate nausea and vomiting after cervical cancer chemotherapy [82].

Constipation and diarrhea persist as major issues for survivors versus healthy controls [83]. More extreme gastrointestinal symptoms correlate with poorer physical and mental health [84]. Colorectal cancer survivors specifically reported high levels of constipation and diarrhea [85]. Physical activity improved diarrhea in prostate cancer survivors [86]. Exercise motivation plans and doctor recommendations together could raise exercise levels in breast and colorectal survivors, potentially improving constipation and diarrhea [87]. Beyond exercise, dietary changes and probiotics have been explored. One study promoted exercise and avoiding sedentary lifestyles for breast cancer survivors [88]. Probiotics during or after cancer treatment may alleviate certain gastrointestinal issues like diarrhea and abdominal pain [89].

3.8 Cardiovascular complications and symptoms in cancer survivors

Cardiovascular complications are a major concern for cancer survivors, as they continue facing increased risk of death from cardiovascular problems after remission or cure [90]. Understanding the mechanisms and diagnostic strategies with risk prediction is key to preventing cardiovascular issues in patients and survivors [91]. Additionally, acquiring modifiable cardiovascular risk factors, especially hypertension, heightens the risk of severe, life-threatening, and fatal cardiac events in survivors, regardless of cancer treatment risks [92]. Long-term cardiovascular effects of cancer treatments like radiotherapy and chemotherapy are well-documented in adult survivors [93]. Furthermore, survivors have high cardiovascular disease risk, with those at risk having significantly higher mortality than those without risk [94]. Preexisting cardiovascular risks and older age associate with heart failure and other cardiovascular diseases in survivors, particularly those who had anthracyclines [95]. Notably, people diagnosed with highly survivable cancers are more likely to die from cardiovascular disease than cancer recurrence, yet cardiovascular risks may be overlooked during survivorship care [96]. This is especially concerning as many breast cancer survivors are more likely to die from cardiovascular disease than breast cancer [97]. Moreover, compared to the general population, survivors have increased risk of cardiovascular events, and the odds of several cardiovascular risk factors are higher among middle-aged survivors [98]. It's estimated cardiovascular disease is the number one comorbidity in survivors and causes many non-cancer deaths among them [99]. Therefore, continuous monitoring and aggressive management of modifiable cardiovascular risks could reduce the cardiovascular burden in cancer survivors.

3.9 Other somatic problems

3.9.1 Osteopenia and osteoporosis in cancer survivors

Osteopenia and osteoporosis are significant concerns for cancer survivors, particularly for breast and prostate cancer survivors. **Table 12** summarizes various mechanisms of bone loss in cancer survivors.

While osteoporosis or osteopenia may seem insignificant compared to other long-term side effects, these disorders can significantly restrict a survivor's lifestyle [100]. Research has shown that younger breast cancer survivors, especially those aged

Factor (s)	Mechanism(s)
Medications	• Glucocorticoids (PO + high dose inhaled) • Excessive thyroid replacement • Proton pump inhibitors • Anticonvulsants • Long-term heparin use • GnRH agonists (Lupron): prostate cancer • Aromatase inhibitors • Thiazolidinediones • Sedative hypnotics (FALL risk) • Furosemide: falls ±calciuresis • Opiates (cause hypogonadism)
Solid tumors	Hypogonadism +/−secondary hyperparathyroid
Various	Weight loss, cachexia
Myeloma	OB inhibition, rarely osteomalacia
Leukemia/lymphoma	Steroids, TKIs
Stem cell transplant	Steroids/GVHD, malabsorption, immunosuppressives, chemo
Neuroendocrine cancer	Ectopic ACTH, Cug syndrome

Table 12.
Etiology of bone loss in cancer patients and survivors.

≤50 years, with estrogen receptor-positive tumors, and those treated with aromatase inhibitors alone or chemotherapy plus any hormone therapy, are at a higher risk for osteopenia and osteoporosis compared to cancer-free women [101]. Adult cancer survivors, including those with childhood leukemia, are also at risk, with approximately 50% of patients having osteopenia or osteoporosis [102]. Similarly, cancer survivors are at risk of developing osteoporosis and osteopenia due to cancer treatment [103]. These conditions often do not produce clinical symptoms until a fracture occurs—commonly seen in the wrist, hip, and spine from minimal trauma that would not typically break a healthy bone. Spinal compression fractures in particular may generate severe back pain, height loss, protruding abdomen, and reduced mobility. More general symptoms can include bone pain, joint aches, and difficulty with walking or daily tasks. Early detection and treatment can reduce fracture risk and related disability.

3.9.2 Respiratory problems in cancer survivors

It is evident that respiratory problems are a significant concern among cancer survivors. Research suggests that childhood cancer survivors had significant excesses in respiratory mortality, including pneumonia, fibrosis, pneumonitis, and other respiratory deaths, with standardized mortality ratios ranging from 7-fold to 17-fold higher than expected [104]. Similarly, highlighted that survivors of childhood and young adult cancer remain at a significantly increased risk of respiratory complications several decades after treatment, emphasizing the importance of clinical initiatives for prevention, early detection, and treatment [105]. Furthermore, reported that adverse health effects, including respiratory infections, were statistically significantly increased in breast cancer survivors, indicating the long-term impact of cancer and its treatment on respiratory health [106]. Additionally, compared the incidence of pulmonary outcomes among cancer survivors and found an increased risk of pulmonary complications, such as asthma, chronic cough, emphysema, lung fibrosis, and recurrent pneumonia, emphasizing the need for ongoing monitoring and management of respiratory health in this population [61].

4. Non-pharmacological approaches to alleviate persistent somatic symptoms

4.1 Physical therapy and rehabilitation

Physical therapy and rehabilitation play a vital role in the care and recovery of cancer survivors. Research has shown that cancer survivors are highly motivated to seek information about physical activity and dietary choices to enhance their response to treatment, expedite recovery, and improve their quality of life [107]. Cancer rehabilitation is a process that helps survivors achieve and maintain the highest possible physical, social, psychological, and vocational functioning within the limits created by cancer and its treatments [108]. In fact, a study evaluating survivors of the 10 most prevalent cancers found that 63% reported the need for at least one rehabilitation service, with physical therapy being the most frequently reported need [109]. Furthermore, investment in oncology physical therapy and the development of international standards of care can allow physical therapists to meet the rehabilitation needs of cancer survivors [110]. Rehabilitation intervention may be required at multiple time points along the cancer continuum, from prior to treatment to the early rehabilitation and long-term survivorship phases post-treatment [111]. Additionally, rehabilitation and exercise have been found to be effective for treating physical functional decline and addressing symptoms across multiple domains and at multiple points along the cancer disease continuum. Moreover, physical activity programs are recommended as part of cancer rehabilitation services [112]. However, there are challenges in implementing physical activity and rehabilitation guidelines in routine primary care cancer rehabilitation, and exploring professionals' perceptions and preparedness to implement these guidelines is essential [113]. Rehabilitation is recommended to help cancer survivors regain functional independence and mitigate subsequent disability [114]. Home exercise programs have been found to be a useful adjunct to physical therapy programs for treating arm and shoulder morbidities in cancer survivors. The American College of Sports Medicine and the American Cancer Society have recommended physical activity as an intervention strategy to help cancer survivors manage symptoms, improve quality of life, and possibly even extend survival [115].

Furthermore, during re-entry after cancer treatment, clinicians can educate survivors on the benefits of healthy behaviors [116]. This period after the primary treatment for cancer ends requires support care for patients having physical, psychological, and social readjustments, making rehabilitation services crucial [117].

4.2 Psychological interventions for somatic symptoms in cancer survivors

Psychological interventions are crucial for addressing the somatic symptoms experienced by cancer survivors. Research shows that cognitive behavioral therapy and physical activity interventions effectively improve quality of life in survivors [118]. Cancer and its treatments can significantly influence psychological well-being and cause distress later in life [24]. Childhood cancer survivors have an increased risk of depression and somatic distress, exacerbated by intensive chemotherapy [18]. Psychological interventions like mindfulness and therapy reduce cancer-related fatigue [26]. Over 35% of survivors experience depressive symptoms during survivorship. Distress manifests as depression, anxiety, PTSD, worry, or anger [27]. Support interventions reduce distress in prostate cancer survivors [25]. Psychosocial interventions increasingly promote resilience and meaning to improve well-being [119, 120]. Disparities in rural survivors' mental health indicate a need to increase their access to services [121]. In summary, a range of psychological interventions are vital to address survivors' somatic symptoms and improve their overall quality of life.

4.3 Integrative therapies for somatic symptoms in cancer survivors

The use of complementary and alternative medicine (CAM) in cancer survivors is widespread and increasing [122]. Certain survivors, like childhood cancer survivors, have high psychological distress, cognitive dysfunction, and poor quality of life [18, 123]. CAM use is high among survivors, but reasons behind use and communication with doctors are not well understood [124]. Many survivors report somatic symptoms and stress. Elderly survivors may have more symptoms, distress, and unhealthy lifestyles [27]. However, lung cancer survivors reported fewer daily somatic symptoms than other survivors [125]. Use of complementary therapies has significantly increased, suggesting survivors are interested in supplementing treatment [126]. Most breast cancer survivors use CAM at some point [127]. Adult survivors of pediatric cancer had more affective, somatic and comorbid symptoms than

DOI: http://dx.doi.org/10.5772/intechopen.1004626

sibling controls [128]. Even long-term survivors use healthcare differently than community controls [129]. Survivors with pain levels similar to people without cancer still engage more in CAM [130]. In summary, CAM use is increasing in survivors and tied to various symptoms, but reasons behind use and impact need further research.

5. Conclusion

Persistent somatic symptoms are highly prevalent in cancer survivors, negatively affecting quality of life across physical, psychological and social domains. Common symptoms include pain, fatigue, sexual dysfunction, cognitive changes, cardiovascular/gastrointestinal issues, respiratory problems, and musculoskeletal disorders. Risk factors like childhood cancer and intensive treatment can worsen burden. Proposed mechanisms involve accelerated aging, somatization, mood disorders, treatment side effects, and physical/psychosocial comorbidities.

Careful assessment of patient-reported outcomes is vital for early detection and management of somatic symptoms. Both drug and non-drug approaches help alleviate persistent symptoms. Evidence-based, patient-centered rehabilitation programs implemented early and continued long-term can significantly mitigate symptoms and improve functioning.

Acknowledgements

I would like to express my sincere gratitude to the faculty members at the Department of Psychiatry, University of Missouri-Kansas City School of Medicine for their guidance and support. Finally, the experiences and struggles of cancer survivors battling persistent somatic and psychological symptoms were the motivation behind this review. I hope my work can positively impact survivorship care and that emerging research continues to alleviate suffering among those courageously recovering from cancer.

Conflict of interest

The authors declares no conflict of interest.

Author details

Val Bellman
Department of Psychiatry, University of Missouri Kansas City School of Medicine, Kansas City, MO, USA

*Address all correspondence to: val.bellmanmd@gmail.com

References

[1] Mandelblatt JS, Zhai W, Ahn J, et al. Symptom burden among older breast cancer survivors: The thinking and living with cancer (TLC) study. Cancer. 2019; **126**:1183-1192

[2] Mao J, Armstrong K, Bowman M, Xie S, Kadakia R, Farrar J. Symptom burden among cancer survivors: Impact of age and comorbidity. The Journal of the American Board of Family Medicine. 2007;**20**(5):434-443. DOI: 10.3122/jabfm.2007.05.060225

[3] Horick N, Muzikansky A, Gutierrez H, Boyd K, Finkelstein D. Physical symptoms in long-term survivors of rare cancer. Journal of Cancer Survivorship. 2018;**12**(6): 835-842. DOI: 10.1007/s11764-018-0721-9

[4] D'Agostino N, Edelstein K, Zhang N, Recklitis C, Brinkman T, Srivastava D, et al. Comorbid symptoms of emotional distress in adult survivors of childhood cancer. Cancer. 2016;**122**(20):3215-3224. DOI: 10.1002/cncr.30171

[5] Zucca A, Boyes A, Linden W, Girgis A. All's well that ends well? Quality of life and physical symptom clusters in long-term cancer survivors across cancer types. Journal of Pain and Symptom Management. 2012;**43**(4): 720-731. DOI: 10.1016/j.jpainsymman.2011.04.023

[6] Leach C, Weaver K, Aziz N, Alfano C, Bellizzi K, Kent E, et al. The complex health profile of long-term cancer survivors: Prevalence and predictors of comorbid conditions. Journal of Cancer Survivorship. 2014; **9**(2):239-251. DOI: 10.1007/s11764-014-0403-1

[7] Cunningham S, Patton M, Schulte F, Richardson P, Heathcote L. Worry about somatic symptoms as a sign of cancer recurrence: Prevalence and associations with fear of recurrence and quality of life in survivors of childhood cancer. Psycho-Oncology. 2021;**30**(7):1077-1085. DOI: 10.1002/pon.5647

[8] Shin H, Dudley W, Bhakta N, Horan M, Wang Z, Bartlett T, et al. Associations of symptom clusters and health outcomes in adult survivors of childhood cancer: A report from the st jude lifetime cohort study. Journal of Clinical Oncology. 2023;**41**(3):497-507. DOI: 10.1200/jco.22.00361

[9] Kroenke K, Zhong X, Theobald D, Wu J, Tu W, Carpenter J. Somatic symptoms in patients with cancer experiencing pain or depression. Archives of Internal Medicine. 2010; **170**(18):1686-1694. DOI: 10.1001/archinternmed.2010.337

[10] Karvonen K, Balay-Dustrude E, Do A, Bradford M, Phipps A, Rosenberg A. Race, ethnicity, and experienced racism are associated with adverse physical and mental health outcomes among cancer survivors. Cancer. 2023;**129**(19):3023-3033. DOI: 10.1002/cncr.34913

[11] Boehmer U, Jesdale B, Streed C, Agénor M. Intersectionality and cancer survivorship: Sexual orientation and racial/ethnic differences in physical and mental health outcomes among female and male cancer survivors. Cancer. 2021; **128**(2):284-291. DOI: 10.1002/cncr.33915

[12] Bernat J, Wittman D, Hawley S, Hamstra D, Helfand A, Haggstrom D, et al. Symptom burden and information needs in prostate cancer survivors: A case for tailored long-term survivorship care. British Journal of Urology. 2015; **118**(3):372-378. DOI: 10.1111/bju.13329

[13] Ness K, Kirkland J, Gramatges M, Wang Z, Kundu M, McCastlain K, et al. Premature physiologic aging as a paradigm for understanding increased risk of adverse health across the lifespan of survivors of childhood cancer. Journal of Clinical Oncology. 2018;**36**(21): 2206-2215. DOI: 10.1200/jco.2017.76.7467

[14] Anderson G, Berk M, Maes M. Biological phenotypes underpin the physio-somatic symptoms of somatization, depression, and chronic fatigue syndrome. Acta Psychiatrica Scandinavica. 2013;**129**(2):83-97. DOI: 10.1111/acps.12182

[15] Chaturvedi S, Maguire G, Somashekar B. Somatization in cancer. International Review of Psychiatry. 2006;**18**(1):49-54. DOI: 10.1080/09540260500466881

[16] Barrineau M, Zarit S, King H, Costanzo E, Almeida D. Daily well-being of cancer survivors: The role of somatic amplification. Psycho-Oncology. 2014; **23**(9):1027-1033. DOI: 10.1002/pon.3509

[17] Michel G, Harju E, Dehler S, Roser K. The long-term impact of cancer: Evaluating psychological distress in adolescent and young adult cancer survivors in Switzerland. Psycho-Oncology. 2019;**28**(3):577-585. DOI: 10.1002/pon.4981

[18] Zebrack B, Zeltzer L, Whitton J, Mertens A, Odom L, Berkow R, et al. Psychological outcomes in long-term survivors of childhood leukemia, hodgkin's disease, and non-hodgkin's lymphoma: A report from the childhood cancer survivor study. Pediatrics. 2002; **110**(1):42-52. DOI: 10.1542/peds.110.1.42

[19] Burghardt J, Klein E, Brähler E, Ernst M, Schneider A, Eckerle S, et al. Prevalence of mental distress among adult survivors of childhood cancer in Germany—Compared to the general population. Cancer Medicine. 2019;**8**(4): 1865-1874. DOI: 10.1002/cam4.1936

[20] Günther M, Schulze J, Jellestad L, Mehnert A, Känel R, Euler S. Mental disorders, length of hospitalization, and psychopharmacy–new approaches to identify barriers to psychological support for patients with cancer. Psycho-Oncology. 2021;**30**(10):1773-1781. DOI: 10.1002/pon.5743

[21] Zheng W, Guo Z. A survey study on the status of somatic symptoms in young and middle-aged patients with mental illness during long-term hospitalization. Contrast Media & Molecular Imaging. 2022;**2022**:1-6. DOI: 10.1155/2022/1110941

[22] Brinkman T, Zhu L, Zeltzer L, Recklitis C, Kimberg C, Zhang N, et al. Longitudinal patterns of psychological distress in adult survivors of childhood cancer. British Journal of Cancer. 2013; **109**(5):1373-1381. DOI: 10.1038/bjc.2013.428

[23] Abdelhadi O, Pollock B, Joseph J, Keegan T. Psychological distress and associated additional medical expenditures in adolescent and young adult cancer survivors. Cancer. 2022; **128**(7):1523-1531. DOI: 10.1002/cncr.34064

[24] Michel G, Rebholz C, Weid N, Bergstraesser E, Kuehni C. Psychological distress in adult survivors of childhood cancer: The swiss childhood cancer survivor study. Journal of Clinical Oncology. 2010;**28**(10):1740-1748. DOI: 10.1200/jco.2009.23.4534

[25] Kamen C, Mustian K, Dozier A, Bowen D, Li Y. Disparities in psychological distress impacting lesbian, gay, bisexual and transgender cancer

survivors. Psycho-Oncology. 2015; **24**(11):1384-1391. DOI: 10.1002/pon.3746

[26] Hovaldt H, Suppli N, Olsen M, Steding-Jessen M, Hansen D, Møller H, et al. Who are the cancer survivors? A nationwide study in Denmark, 1943–2010. British Journal of Cancer. 2015; **112**(9):1549-1553. DOI: 10.1038/bjc.2015.68

[27] Grov E, Fossa S, Dahl A. Is somatic comorbidity associated with more somatic symptoms, mental distress, or unhealthy lifestyle in elderly cancer survivors? Journal of Cancer Survivorship. 2009;**3**(2):109-116. DOI: 10.1007/s11764-009-0081-6

[28] Heathcote L, Loecher N, Simon P, Spunt S, Jordan A, Tutelman P, et al. Symptom appraisal in uncertainty: A theory-driven thematic analysis with survivors of childhood cancer. Psychology and Health. 2020;**36**(10): 1182-1199. DOI: 10.1080/08870446.2020.1836180

[29] Tuman M, Roberts K, Corner G, Beard C, Fadalla C, Coats T, et al. Interpretation bias in breast cancer survivors experiencing fear of cancer recurrence. Frontiers in Psychology. 2021;**12**:682174. DOI: 10.3389/fpsyg.2021.682174

[30] Hall D, Lennes I, Pirl W, Friedman E, Park E. Fear of recurrence or progression as a link between somatic symptoms and perceived stress among cancer survivors. Supportive Care in Cancer. 2016;**25**(5):1401-1407

[31] Lowery A, Starr T, Dhingra L, Rogak L, Hamrick-Price J, Farberov M, et al. Frequency, characteristics, and correlates of pain in a pilot study of colorectal cancer survivors 1–10 years post-treatment. Pain Medicine. 2013; **14**(11):1673-1680. DOI: 10.1111/pme.12223

[32] Yang M, Baser R, Li S, Hou Y, Chong K, Zhang Y, et al. Tibetan herbal pain-relieving plaster for chronic musculoskeletal pain among cancer survivors: Study protocol of a randomized, double-blind, placebo-controlled trial. Frontiers in Pharmacology. 2022;**13**:878371. DOI: 10.3389/fphar.2022.878371

[33] Marshall V, Chavez M, Efre A, Lake P, Rigg K, Lubrano B, et al. Barriers to adequate pain control and opioid use among cancer survivors: Implications for nursing practice. Cancer Nursing. 2022; **46**(5):386-393. DOI: 10.1097/ncc.0000000000001126

[34] Check D, Jones K, Fish L, Dinan M, Dunbar T, Farley S, et al. Clinician perspectives on managing chronic pain after curative-intent cancer treatment. Jco Oncology Practice. 2023;**19**(4):e484-e491. DOI: 10.1200/op.22.00410

[35] O'Regan A, Fish L, Makarushka C, Somers T, Jones K, Merlin J, et al. Managing chronic pain in cancer survivorship: Communication challenges and opportunities as described by cancer survivors. The American Journal of Hospice & Palliative Care. 2022;**41**(1): 78-86. DOI: 10.21203/rs.3.rs-2221806/v1

[36] Sanford N, Sher D, Butler S, Xu X, Ahn C, Aizer A, et al. Prevalence of chronic pain among cancer survivors in the United States, 2010-2017. Cancer. 2019;**125**(23):4310-4318. DOI: 10.1002/cncr.32450

[37] Stein K, Alcaraz K, Kamson C, Fallon E, Smith T. Sociodemographic inequalities in barriers to cancer pain management: A report from the american cancer society's study of cancer survivors-ii (scs-ii). Psycho-Oncology.

2016;**25**(10):1212-1221. DOI: 10.1002/pon.4218

[38] Mercadante S, Grassi Y, Gebbia V. Cancer survivors: Long-term opioid therapy – The challenge. BMJ Supportive & Palliative Care. 2022;**14**(1):65-67. DOI: 10.1136/spcare-2022-003974

[39] Jones K, Magee L, Fu M, Bernacki R, Bulls H, Merlin J, et al. The contribution of cancer-specific psychosocial factors to the pain experience in cancer survivors. Journal of Hospice and Palliative Nursing. 2023;**25**(5):E85-E93. DOI: 10.1097/njh.0000000000000965

[40] Drury A, Payne S, Brady A. The cost of survival: An exploration of colorectal cancer survivors' experiences of pain. Acta Oncologica. 2017;**56**(2):205-211. DOI: 10.1080/0284186x.2016.1266084

[41] Mao J, Liou K, Baser R, Bao T, Panageas K, Romero S, et al. Effectiveness of electroacupuncture or auricular acupuncture vs usual care for chronic musculoskeletal pain among cancer survivors. JAMA Oncology. 2021; **7**(5):720. DOI: 10.1001/jamaoncol.2021.0310

[42] Wang H, Liu X, Wang T, Tan J, Huang H. Breathing exercises for pain management in cancer survivors: A systematic review. Pain Management Nursing. 2022;**24**(3):299-310. DOI: 10.20944/preprints202203.0156.v1

[43] Tofthagen C, González L, Visovsky C, Akers A. Self-management of oxaliplatin-related peripheral neuropathy in colorectal cancer survivors. Chemotherapy Research and Practice. 2013;**2013**:1-7. DOI: 10.1155/2013/547932

[44] Kim S, Son B, Hwang S, Han W, Yang J, Lee S, et al. Fatigue and depression in disease-free breast cancer survivors: Prevalence, correlates, and association with quality of life. Journal of Pain and Symptom Management. 2008; **35**(6):644-655. DOI: 10.1016/j.jpainsymman.2007.08.012

[45] Wang X, Zhao F, Fisch M, O'Mara A, Cella D, Mendoza T, et al. Prevalence and characteristics of moderate to severe fatigue: A multicenter study in cancer patients and survivors. Cancer. 2013;**120**(3):425-432. DOI: 10.1002/cncr.28434

[46] Pachman D, Barton D, Swetz K, Loprinzi C. Troublesome symptoms in cancer survivors: Fatigue, insomnia, neuropathy, and pain. Journal of Clinical Oncology. 2012;**30**(30):3687-3696. DOI: 10.1200/jco.2012.41.7238

[47] Yu C, Wang T, Chang C, Shen L, Shu W, Liu C, et al. Healthy life styles, sleep and fatigue in endometrial cancer survivors: A cross-sectional study. Journal of Clinical Nursing. 2020;**29**(7–8):1372-1380. DOI: 10.1111/jocn.15189

[48] Daniëls L, Oerlemans S, Krol A, Creutzberg C, Poll-Franse L. Chronic fatigue in hodgkin lymphoma survivors and associations with anxiety, depression and comorbidity. British Journal of Cancer. 2014;**110**(4):868-874. DOI: 10.1038/bjc.2013.779

[49] Gielissen M, Verhagen S, Witjes F, Bleijenberg G. Effects of cognitive behavior therapy in severely fatigued disease-free cancer patients compared with patients waiting for cognitive behavior therapy: A randomized controlled trial. Journal of Clinical Oncology. 2006;**24**(30):4882-4887. DOI: 10.1200/jco.2006.06.8270

[50] Oktay J, Bellin M, Scarvalone S, Appling S, Helzlsouer K. Managing the impact of posttreatment fatigue on the family: Breast cancer survivors share

their experiences. Families, Systems & Health. 2011;**29**(2):127-137. DOI: 10.1037/a0023947

[51] Sprod L, Fernandez I, Janelsins M, Peppone L, Atkins J, Giguere J, et al. Effects of yoga on cancer-related fatigue and global side-effect burden in older cancer survivors. Journal of Geriatric Oncology. 2015;**6**(1):8-14. DOI: 10.1016/j.jgo.2014.09.184

[52] Ikeuchi K, Ishiguro H, Nakamura Y, Izawa T, Kura N, Nin K. The relation between mindfulness and the fatigue of women with breast cancer: Path analysis. Biopsychosocial Medicine. 2020;**14**(1). DOI: 10.1186/s13030-020-0175-y. Available from: https://www.ncbi.nlm.nih.gov/pmc/articles/PMC7011601/

[53] Peixoto T, Peixoto N, Santos C, Pinto C. Fatigue self-management strategies in cancer survivors: A systematic literature review. Revista De Enfermagem Referência. 2016;**IV Série**(10):113-124. DOI: 10.12707/riv16023

[54] Prasad P, Hardy K, Zhang N, Edelstein K, Srivastava D, Zeltzer L, et al. Psychosocial and neurocognitive outcomes in adult survivors of adolescent and early young adult cancer: A report from the childhood cancer survivor study. Journal of Clinical Oncology. 2015;**33**(23):2545-2552. DOI: 10.1200/jco.2014.57.7528

[55] Ah D, Storey S, Tallman E, Nielsen A, Johns S, Pressler S. Cancer, cognitive impairment, and work-related outcomes: An integrative review. Oncology Nursing Forum. 2016;**43**(5):602-616. DOI: 10.1188/16.onf.602-616

[56] John T, Sender L, Bota D. Cognitive impairment in survivors of adolescent and early young adult onset non-cns cancers: Does chemotherapy play a role? Journal of Adolescent and Young Adult Oncology. 2016;**5**(3):226-231. DOI: 10.1089/jayao.2015.0025

[57] Phillips N, Stratton K, Williams A, Ahles T, Ness K, Cohen H, et al. Late-onset cognitive impairment and modifiable risk factors in adult childhood cancer survivors. JAMA Network Open. 2023;**6**(5):e2316077. DOI: 10.1001/jamanetworkopen.2023.16077

[58] Cherrier M, Anderson K, David D, Higano C, Gray H, Church A, et al. A randomized trial of cognitive rehabilitation in cancer survivors. Life Sciences. 2013;**93**(17):617-622. DOI: 10.1016/j.lfs.2013.08.011

[59] Barlow-Krelina E, Chen Y, Yasui Y, Till C, Gibson T, Ness K, et al. Consistent physical activity and future neurocognitive problems in adult survivors of childhood cancers: A report from the childhood cancer survivor study. Journal of Clinical Oncology. 2020;**38**(18):2041-2052. DOI: 10.1200/jco.19.02677

[60] Haque R, Hsu JW, Avila C, Olmstead R, Carroll JE, Irwin MR. Insomnia and susceptibility to depressive symptoms and fatigue in diverse breast cancer survivors. Journal of Women's Health (2002). 2021;**30**(11):1604-1615. DOI: 10.1089/jwh.2019.8135

[61] Dietz AC, Chen Y, Yasui Y, et al. Risk and impact of pulmonary complications in survivors of childhood cancer: A report from the childhood cancer survivor study. Cancer. 2016;**122**(23):3687-3696. DOI: 10.1002/cncr.30200

[62] Schlarb AA, Claßen M, Hellmann SM, Vögele C, Gulewitsch MD. Sleep and somatic complaints in university students. Journal of Pain Research. 2017;**10**:1189-1199. DOI: 10.2147/JPR.S125421

[63] Wei Y, Blanken TF, Van Someren EJW. Insomnia really hurts: Effect of a bad night's sleep on pain increases with insomnia severity. Frontiers in Psychiatry. 2018;**9**:377. DOI: 10.3389/fpsyt.2018.00377

[64] Sun Y, Wang L, Li C, Luo W. Sleep disturbance in Chinese college students with mental health problems: A moderated mediation model. International Journal of Environmental Research and Public Health. 2022;**19**(21): 14570. DOI: 10.3390/ijerph192114570

[65] Cherven B, Sampson A, Bober S, Bingen K, Frederick N, Freyer D, et al. Sexual health among adolescent and young adult cancer survivors: A scoping review from the children's oncology group adolescent and young adult oncology discipline committee. CA a Cancer Journal for Clinicians. 2020;**71**(3):250-263. DOI: 10.3322/caac.21655

[66] Ford J, Kawashima T, Whitton J, Leisenring W, Laverdière C, Stovall M, et al. Psychosexual functioning among adult female survivors of childhood cancer: A report from the childhood cancer survivor study. Journal of Clinical Oncology. 2014;**32**(28):3126-3136. DOI: 10.1200/jco.2013.54.1086

[67] Bjornard K, Howell C, Klosky J, Chemaitilly W, Srivastava D, Brinkman T, et al. Psychosexual functioning of female childhood cancer survivors: A report from the st. jude lifetime cohort study. Journal of Sexual Medicine. 2020;**17**(10):1981-1994. DOI: 10.1016/j.jsxm.2020.06.005

[68] Hovén E, Fagerkvist K, Jahnukainen K, Ljungman L, Lähteenmäki P, Axelsson O, et al. Sexual dysfunction in young adult survivors of childhood cancer – A population-based study. European Journal of Cancer. 2021;**154**:147-156. DOI: 10.1016/j.ejca.2021.06.014

[69] Ritenour C, Seidel K, Leisenring W, Mertens A, Wasilewski-Masker K, Shnorhavorian M, et al. Erectile dysfunction in male survivors of childhood cancer—A report from the childhood cancer survivor study. Journal of Sexual Medicine. 2016;**13**(6):945-954. DOI: 10.1016/j.jsxm.2016.03.367

[70] El-Hosary E, Abd-Elsalam A. Effect of standard oncology nursing care intervention on reducing "sexual dysfunction" among cervical cancer survivors' women. Nursing & Primary Care. 2018;**2**(4):1-7. DOI: 10.33425/2639-9474.1072

[71] Maass S, Boerman L, Brandenbarg D, Verhaak P, Maduro J, Bock G, et al. Symptoms in long-term breast cancer survivors: A cross-sectional study in primary care. The Breast. 2020;**54**: 133-138. DOI: 10.1016/j.breast.2020.09.013

[72] Schlairet M, Benton M. Quality of life and perceived educational needs among older cancer survivors. Journal of Cancer Education. 2011;**27**(1):21-26. DOI: 10.1007/s13187-011-0279-y

[73] Sari N. Physical wellbeing in cervical and breast cancer survivors: A cross-sectional study in Surabaya, Indonesia. Indonesian Journal of Cancer. 2019; **12**(3):80. DOI: 10.33371/ijoc.v12i3.614

[74] Jackson S, Williams K, Steptoe A, Wardle J. The impact of a cancer diagnosis on weight change: Findings from prospective, population-based cohorts in the UK and the US. BMC Cancer. 2014;**14**(1):926. DOI: 10.1186/1471-2407-14-926

[75] Nho J, Kim S, Park M, Kweon S. Symptom clusters and quality of life in breast cancer survivors after cancer treatment in a tertiary hospital in Korea.

European Journal of Cancer Care. 2018; **27**(6):e12919. DOI: 10.1111/ecc.12919

[76] May C, Ho A, Yang Q, McCallum M, Iyengar N, Comander A, et al. Comparing outcomes of a digital commercial weight loss program in adult cancer survivors and matched controls with overweight or obesity: Retrospective analysis. Nutrients. 2021; **13**(9):2908. DOI: 10.3390/nu13092908

[77] Naeim A, Dy S, Lorenz K, Sanati H, Walling A, Asch S. Evidence-based recommendations for cancer nausea and vomiting. Journal of Clinical Oncology. 2008;**26**(23):3903-3910. DOI: 10.1200/jco.2007.15.9533

[78] Roiland R, Heidrich S. Symptom clusters and quality of life in older adult breast cancer survivors. Oncology Nursing Forum. 2011;**38**(6):672-680. DOI: 10.1188/11.onf.672-680

[79] Wood G, Lynch B, Roenn J. Management of intractable nausea and vomiting in patients at the end of life. JAMA. 2007;**298**(10):1196. DOI: 10.1001/jama.298.10.1196

[80] Puspita Z, Nissa C, Probosari E, Fitranti D. Consumption pattern score in cancer survivor with chemotherapy induced nausea and vomiting and non-cancer at shelter houses. Jurnal Gizi Indonesia (The Indonesian Journal of Nutrition). 2022;**11**(1):57-65. DOI: 10.14710/jgi.11.1.57-65

[81] Taşpınar A, Şirin A. Effect of acupressure on chemotherapy-induced nausea and vomiting in gynecologic cancer patients in Turkey. European Journal of Oncology Nursing. 2010; **14**(1):49-54. DOI: 10.1016/j.ejon.2009.07.006

[82] Sriningsih I, Elisa E, Lestari K. Aromatherapy ginger use in patients with nausea & vomiting on post cervical cancer chemotherapy. Jurnal Kesehatan Masyarakat. 2017;**13**(1):59-68. DOI: 10.15294/kemas.v13i1.5367

[83] Thong M, Doege D, Weißer L, Jansen L, Bertram H, Eberle A, et al. Persisting deficits in health-related quality of life of colorectal cancer survivors 14–24 years post-diagnosis: A population-based study. Current Oncology. 2023;**30**(3):3373-3390. DOI: 10.3390/curroncol30030257

[84] Deleemans J, Toivonen K, Reimer R, Carlson L. The chemo-gut study: A cross-sectional survey exploring physical, mental, and gastrointestinal health outcomes in cancer survivors. Global Advances in Health and Medicine. 2022;**11**. DOI: 10.1177/2164957x221145940. Available from: https://pubmed.ncbi.nlm.nih.gov/36583068/

[85] Tang F, Wang J, Tang Z, Kang M, Deng Q, Yu J. Quality of life and its association with physical activity among different types of cancer survivors. PLoS One. 2016;**11**(11):e0164971. DOI: 10.1371/journal.pone.0164971

[86] Zhuang J, Liu Y, Xu X, Cai Y, Liu M, Chen Z, et al. Association between physical activity and health-related quality of life: Time to deterioration model analysis in lung adenocarcinoma. Journal of Cancer Survivorship. 2022; **17**(6):1769-1779. DOI: 10.1007/s11764-022-01259-z

[87] Park J, Lee J, Oh M, Park H, Chae J, Kim D, et al. The effect of oncologists' exercise recommendations on the level of exercise and quality of life in survivors of breast and colorectal cancer: A randomized controlled trial. Cancer. 2015;**121**(16):2740-2748. DOI: 10.1002/cncr.29400

[88] Barchitta M, Maugeri A, Lio R, Quattrocchi A, Degrassi F, Catalano F, et al. The effects of diet and dietary interventions on the quality of life among breast cancer survivors: A cross-sectional analysis and a systematic review of experimental studies. Cancers. 2020;**12**(2):322. DOI: 10.3390/cancers12020322

[89] Deleemans J, Gajtani Z, Baydoun M, Reimer R, Piedalue K, Carlson L. The use of prebiotic and probiotic interventions for treating gastrointestinal and psychosocial health symptoms in cancer patients and survivors: A systematic review. Integrative Cancer Therapies. 2021;**20**. DOI: 10.1177/153473542 11061733. Available from: https://www.ncbi.nlm.nih.gov/pmc/articles/PMC8649088/

[90] Mohammed T, Parekh T, Desai A. Cardiovascular risk management in cancer survivors: Are we doing it right? World Journal of Clinical Oncology. 2021;**12**(3):144-149. DOI: 10.5306/wjco.v12.i3.144

[91] Kadowaki H, Akazawa H, Ishida J, Komuro I. Cancer therapeutics-related cardiac dysfunction — Insights from bench and bedside of onco-cardiology. Circulation Journal. 2020;**84**(9): 1446-1453. DOI: 10.1253/circj.cj-20-0467

[92] Armstrong G, Oeffinger K, Chen Y, Kawashima T, Yasui Y, Leisenring W, et al. Modifiable risk factors and major cardiac events among adult survivors of childhood cancer. Journal of Clinical Oncology. 2013;**31**(29):3673-3680. DOI: 10.1200/jco.2013.49.3205

[93] Naaktgeboren W, Linschoten M, Graeff A, Rhenen A, Asselbergs F, Maas A, et al. Long-term cardiovascular health in adult cancer survivors. Maturitas. 2017;**105**:37-45. DOI: 10.1016/j.maturitas.2017.05.014

[94] Lee S, Cartmell K. An association rule mining analysis of lifestyle behavioral risk factors in cancer survivors with high cardiovascular disease risk. Journal of Personalized Medicine. 2021;**11**(5):366. DOI: 10.3390/jpm11050366

[95] Salz T, Zabor E, Brown P, Dalton S, Raghunathan N, Matasar M, et al. Preexisting cardiovascular risk and subsequent heart failure among non-hodgkin lymphoma survivors. Journal of Clinical Oncology. 2017;**35**(34): 3837-3843. DOI: 10.1200/jco.2017.72.4211

[96] Weaver K, Foraker R, Alfano C, Rowland J, Arora N, Bellizzi K, et al. Cardiovascular risk factors among long-term survivors of breast, prostate, colorectal, and gynecologic cancers: A gap in survivorship care? Journal of Cancer Survivorship. 2013;7(2):253-261. DOI: 10.1007/s11764-013-0267-9

[97] Weaver K, Klepin H, Wells B, Dressler E, Winkfield K, Lamar Z, et al. Cardiovascular assessment tool for breast cancer survivors and oncology providers: Usability study. Jmir Cancer. 2021;7(1):e18396. DOI: 10.2196/18396

[98] Loreti C, Castelli L, Coraci D, Fusco A, Giovannini S, Padua L. Polipharmacy and multimorbity in oncological patients: An open challenge. Current Oncology. 2021;**28**(1):273-274. DOI: 10.3390/curroncol28010030

[99] Schoormans D, Vissers P, Herk-Sukel M, Denollet J, Pedersen S, Dalton S, et al. Incidence of cardiovascular disease up to 13 year after cancer diagnosis: A matched cohort study among 32,757 cancer survivors. Cancer Medicine. 2018;7(10):4952-4963. DOI: 10.1002/cam4.1754

[100] Rodgers C, Monroe R. Osteopenia and osteoporosis in pediatric patients after stem cell transplant. Journal of Pediatric Oncology Nursing. 2007;**24**(4): 184-189. DOI: 10.1177/1043454207303942

[101] Ramin C, May B, Roden R, Orellana M, Hogan B, McCullough M, et al. Evaluation of osteopenia and osteoporosis in younger breast cancer survivors compared with cancer-free women: A prospective cohort study. Breast Cancer Research. 2018;**20**(1):134. DOI: 10.1186/s13058-018-1061-4

[102] Choi Y, Park S, Cho W, Lee J, Hahn S, Jung M, et al. Factors related to decreased bone mineral density in childhood cancer survivors. Journal of Korean Medical Science. 2013;**28**(11): 1632. DOI: 10.3346/jkms.2013.28.11.1632

[103] Hershman D, Narayanan R. Prevention and management of osteoporosis in women with breast cancer and men with prostate cancer. Current Oncology Reports. 2004;**6**(4): 277-284. DOI: 10.1007/s11912-004-0036-z

[104] Fidler M, Reulen R, Bright C, Henson K, Kelly J, Jenney M, et al. Respiratory mortality of childhood, adolescent and young adult cancer survivors. Thorax. 2018;**73**(10):959-968. DOI: 10.1136/thoraxjnl-2017-210683

[105] Smith G, Glaser A, Peckham D, Greenwood D, Feltbower R. Respiratory morbidity in young people surviving cancer: Population-based study of hospital admissions, treatment-related risk factors and subsequent mortality. International Journal of Cancer. 2019;**145**(1):20-28. DOI: 10.1002/ijc.32066

[106] Heins M, Ligt K, Verloop J, Siesling S, Korevaar J, Berendsen A, et al. Adverse health effects after breast cancer up to 14 years after diagnosis. The Breast. 2022;**61**:22-28. DOI: 10.1016/j.breast.2021.12.001

[107] Rock C, Doyle C, Demark-Wahnefried W, Meyerhardt J, Courneya K, Schwartz A, et al. Nutrition and physical activity guidelines for cancer survivors. CA a Cancer Journal for Clinicians. 2012;**62**(4):242-274. DOI: 10.3322/caac.21142

[108] Stubblefield M. The underutilization of rehabilitation to treat physical impairments in breast cancer survivors. PM & R. 2017;**9**(9S2):S317-S323. DOI: 10.1016/j.pmrj.2017.05.010

[109] Silver J, Baima J, Mayer R. Impairment-driven cancer rehabilitation: An essential component of quality care and survivorship. CA A Cancer Journal for Clinicians. 2013; **63**(5):295-317. DOI: 10.3322/caac.21186

[110] Brennan L, Sheill G, O'Neill L, O'Connor L, Smyth E, Guinan E. Physical therapists in oncology settings: Experiences in delivering cancer rehabilitation services, barriers to care, and service development needs. Physical Therapy. 2022;**102**(3):pzab287. DOI: 10.1093/ptj/pzab287

[111] Dunphy C, McNeely M. Growing the workforce in oncology physical therapy: From entry level to specialist care. Rehabilitation Oncology. 2022; **40**(1):5-6. DOI: 10.1097/01.reo.0000000000000277

[112] Rossen S, Kayser L, Vibe-Petersen J, Christensen J, Ried-Larsen M. Cancer survivors' receptiveness to digital technology–supported physical rehabilitation and the implications for design: Qualitative study. Journal of Medical Internet Research. 2020;**22**(8): e15335. DOI: 10.2196/15335

[113] Neher M, Ludvigsson M, Enblom A. Preparedness to implement physical activity and rehabilitation guidelines in routine primary care cancer rehabilitation: Focus group interviews exploring rehabilitation professionals' perceptions. Journal of Cancer Education. 2020;**36**(4):779-786. DOI: 10.1007/s13187-020-01704-6

[114] Rafn B, Midtgaard J, Camp P, Campbell K. Shared concern with current breast cancer rehabilitation services: A focus group study of survivors' and professionals' experiences and preferences for rehabilitation care delivery. BMJ Open. 2020;**10**(7): e037280. DOI: 10.1136/bmjopen-2020-037280

[115] Courneya K, Rogers L, Campbell K, Vallance J, Friedenreich C. Top 10 research questions related to physical activity and cancer survivorship. Research Quarterly for Exercise and Sport. 2015;**86**(2):107-116. DOI: 10.1080/02701367.2015.991265

[116] Troeschel A, Leach C, Shuval K, Stein K, Patel A. Physical activity in cancer survivors during "re-entry" following cancer treatment. Preventing Chronic Disease. 2018;**15**:E65. DOI: 10.5888/pcd15.170277

[117] Kang J, Park E, Lee J. Cancer survivorship in primary care. Korean Journal of Family Medicine. 2019;**40**(6): 353-361. DOI: 10.4082/kjfm.19.0108

[118] Weaver K, Forsythe L, Reeve B, Alfano C, Rodriguez J, Sabatino S, et al. Mental and physical health–related quality of life among U.S. cancer survivors: Population estimates from the 2010 national health interview survey. Cancer Epidemiology Biomarkers & Prevention. 2012;**21**(11):2108-2117. DOI: 10.1158/1055-9965.epi-12-0740

[119] Holtmaat K, Spek N, Lissenberg-Witte B, Cuijpers P, Leeuw I. Positive mental health among cancer survivors: Overlap in psychological well-being, personal meaning, and posttraumatic growth. Supportive Care in Cancer. 2018;**27**(2):443-450. DOI: 10.1007/s00520-018-4325-8

[120] Harms C, Cohen L, Pooley J, Chambers S, Galvão D, Newton R. Quality of life and psychological distress in cancer survivors: The role of psycho-social resources for resilience. Psycho-Oncology. 2018;**28**(2):271-277. DOI: 10.1002/pon.4934

[121] Burris J, Andrykowski M. Disparities in mental health between rural and nonrural cancer survivors: A preliminary study. Psycho-Oncology. 2009;**19**(6):637-645. DOI: 10.1002/pon.1600

[122] Adams M, Jewell A. The use of complementary and alternative medicine by cancer patients. International Seminars in Surgical Oncology. 2007;**4**(1):655-663. DOI: 10.1186/1477-7800-4-10

[123] Zeltzer L, Recklitis C, Buchbinder D, Zebrack B, Casillas J, Tsao J, et al. Psychological status in childhood cancer survivors: A report from the childhood cancer survivor study. Journal of Clinical Oncology. 2009;**27**(14):2396-2404. DOI: 10.1200/jco.2008.21.1433

[124] Mao J, Palmer C, Healy K, Desai K, Amsterdam J. Complementary and alternative medicine use among cancer survivors: A population-based study. Journal of Cancer Survivorship. 2010; **5**(1):8-17. DOI: 10.1007/s11764-010-0153-7

[125] Aronson K, Wagstaff D, Farace E, Muscat J, Belani C, Almokadem S, et al. A week in the life of lung cancer

survivors: Daily reports of stress, worry, mood, and symptoms. Journal of Health Psychology. 2016;**21**(10):2269-2282. DOI: 10.1177/1359105315574921

[126] Husebø A, Husebø T. Quality of life and breast cancer: How can mind–body exercise therapies help? An overview study. Sports. 2017;**5**(4):79. DOI: 10.3390/sports5040079

[127] Slocum-Gori S, Howard A, Balneaves L, Kazanjian A. Investigating the perceived feasibility of integrative medicine in a conventional oncology setting. Integrative Cancer Therapies. 2012;**12**(2):103-112. DOI: 10.1177/1534735412443851

[128] Barone R, Gulisano M, Cannata E, Padalino S, Saia F, Maugeri N, et al. Self- and parent-reported psychological symptoms in young cancer survivors and control peers: Results from a clinical center. Journal of Clinical Medicine. 2020;**9**(11):3444. DOI: 10.3390/jcm9113444

[129] Nord C, Mykletun A, Thorsen L, Bjøro T, Fosså S. Self-reported health and use of health care services in long-term cancer survivors. International Journal of Cancer. 2004;**114**(2):307-316. DOI: 10.1002/ijc.20713

[130] Fouladbakhsh J, Stommel M. Comparative analysis of cam use in the U.S. cancer and noncancer populations. Journal of Complementary and Integrative Medicine. 2008;**5**(1):9-10. DOI: 10.2202/1553-3840.1140

Chapter 5

Management of Body Dysmorphic Disorder in Dermatology Cosmetic

Dian Andriani Ratna Dewi, Amin Ibrizatun, Lila Irawati Tjahjo Widuri, Hayra Avianggi and Fakhira Ayu Wijayanti

Abstract

Somatic symptom disorder is prevalent in patients in various medical specializations, primary healthcare settings, and the general public. One psychiatric diagnosis that falls within the category of obsessive-compulsive disorder and related disorders is body dysmorphic disorder. The patient is fixated on a minor, imaginary defect in their look. The patient magnifies even the slightest irregularities, which causes them to feel guilty and embarrassed and has a detrimental effect on their lives. Patients with body dysmorphic disorder were more common in general care and dermatology clinics than in psychiatric settings. It is not, however, a commonly recognized idea in dermatologists' daily clinical practice. Body dysmorphic disorder, a somatoform disorder also referred to as dysmorphophobia, is a non-dermatological condition that is frequently misdiagnosed and goes untreated.

Keywords: somatic symptom disorder, body dysmorphic disorder, dysmorphophobia, obsessive-compulsive disorder, imaginary defect

1. Introduction

Somatic symptom disorder (SSD) is defined by the Diagnostic and Statistical Manual of Mental Disorders, Fifth Edition (DSM-V) as the co-existence of one or more physical symptoms and excessive time, energy, emotions, and behavior associated with a mental illness. These symptoms may or may not be connected to a health issue. Research has looked at risk factors such as chaotic living, early maltreatment, sexual assault, and a history of alcohol and drug misuse, even though the exact cause of SSD is still unknown. Axis II personality disorders, such as avoidant, paranoid, self-defeating, and obsessive-compulsive, have also been linked to significant somatization. Psychosocial stressors are also connected to poor job performance and unemployment [1].

2. Types of somatic symptom disorder

2.1 Somatoform disorder

Recurrent subjective feelings of physical symptoms (hereafter referred to as somatoform symptoms) that are not related to any physical disease are characteristic of somatoform diseases. Physical abnormalities alone cannot explain the type and severity of somatoform symptoms. Children with attention-seeking behavior are often affected [2]. A systematic study of studies in 24 countries found that the prevalence of somatoform diseases varied from 26.2 to 34.8% among primary care patients [3].

Stress is often a predisposing factor for somatoform disorders, acting as a trigger and cause of their development. Persistent symptoms of somatoform disease may be related to a person's personality, early life experiences (difficulties faced during childhood), events encountered, persistent stress, coping mechanisms (inability to handle the demands of daily life), unhealthy lifestyle (abuse drugs, inactivity, irregular sleep patterns), can be accompanied by medical or psychological disorders and can also be cultural factors [4].

Short-term goals of the treatment of somatoform disorder are to reduce symptoms, stop increasingly useless medical procedures, maintain a reasonable level of medical care, and initiate activities appropriate to the patient's age. The long-term goal is to be able to return to age-appropriate activities, be able to manage psychological and environmental stressors and provide appropriate—not excessive—medical care [4].

2.2 Hypochondriasis

According to the International Classification of Diseases, 10th Edition (ICD-10), hypochondriasis is a distinct disease characterized by obsession with the possibility of one or more severe and progressive bodily disorders. ICD-10 and DSM-4 classify this disease as a somatoform disorder. ICD-10 includes body dysmorphic disorder, which falls into the category of hypochondriac disease. The DSM-5 classifies hypochondriasis as an illness anxiety disorder (IAD) and puts it in the category of somatic symptoms and related disorders. According to reports, the prevalence of hypochondriasis ranges from 0.8 to 8.5% in primary care studies and between 0.02% and 7% in general population studies [5].

Treatment for this disease includes [2]:

First line: Cognitive Behavioral Therapy (CBT) for restructuring cognition, exposing oneself, and preventing reactions to address maladaptive behavior.

Second line: Mindfulness-Based Cognitive Therapy (MBCT) integrates aspects of CBT with mindfulness meditation. Acceptance as well as commitment therapy includes commitment to changing behavior, acceptance of frightened thoughts and feelings, mindfulness training, and value clarification.

Third line: Before putting prospective solutions into action, problem resolution therapy includes recognizing, describing, and weighing them. Treatments for relaxation include diaphragmatic breathing, progressive muscle relaxation, and release-only muscle relaxation. Time management, assertiveness training, problem-solving, and relaxation techniques are all incorporated into behavioral stress management.

2.3 Illness anxiety disorder

IAD is a psychiatric disease defined by excessive anxiety that one may have or acquire as a significant medical problem that is untreated. The name hypochondriasis was previously used but was updated in the DSM-5 due to its derogatory implications. People with IAD experience persistent worry or anxiety that is connected to a significant medical condition and interferes with their daily functioning. Even when the laboratory findings and physical examinations are normal, this worry nevertheless exists. Individuals with IAD mistakenly perceive bodily sensations like sweating or digestion as signs of a serious illness, leading them to overanalyze these experiences. IAD is typically a long-term illness. IAD sufferers may feel uneasy experiencing typical bodily feelings and they might diagnose little alterations in the body as abnormal. IAD may arise if a person is raised in a home where health issues are regularly mentioned or if their parents worry excessively about their well-being [6].

When given a negative diagnosis, patients with IAD typically do not feel satisfied and see several doctors for the same illness. They thought that their prior physician was incompetent, inattentive, or ignored their significant medical condition, which could have had deleterious results. Most IAD patients fit into one of two categories [6, 7]: 1. care-seeking type. These patients regularly switch doctors and take advantage of the healthcare system. They might ask for multiple tests and procedures. 2. avoidant of care. These people stay away from doctors. They are highly anxious and worried that either their primary care physician or laboratory tests will reveal a life-threatening condition (such as cancer). A general medical problem does not make an IAD diagnosis impossible.

Helping patients with illnesses or anxiety disorders overcome their health anxiety is the primary objective of their treatment. It is important to acknowledge the patient's worries and anxieties. Avoid sayings such as "it is all in your head." Patients may be referred to additional medical professionals as needed. Excessive use of medical systems, pointless imaging investigations, expert referrals, and laboratory testing should be avoided once major medical diseases have been ruled out and an IAD diagnosis has been made. Patients should make an appointment for routine follow-up visits with both their psychiatrist and primary care provider. Regular follow-up will cut down on emergency room or other physician visits. Additionally, the physician can critically evaluate new symptoms and related stresses and triggers. The initial course of treatment for IAD is psychotherapy. Behavior modification techniques are used in CBT, a form of psychotherapy, to correct a patient's dysfunctional, maladaptive cognitive beliefs. This could help with the patient's excessive body inspection habit for disease indicators [6].

Pharmacological treatments are the second-line therapy for IAD. Antidepressants, such as selective serotonin reuptake inhibitors (SSRI) and serotonin norepinephrine reuptake inhibitors (SNRI), are effective in treating this disorder. Patients who respond well to antidepressant therapy are encouraged to stay on maintenance care for a minimum of 6–12 months. Most individuals require both medicine and psychotherapy at the same time [8].

2.4 Body dysmorphic disorder

Body dysmorphic disorder (BDD), or dysmorphophobia, is defined by the DSM-5 as an obsession with perceived physical appearance problems that are invisible to others or very slightly noticeable. One's ability to function in social, intellectual, professional, and other arenas is severely hampered by this fixation since it is so strong. These behaviors usually take a long time, are challenging to cease, and upset the person. An average of 3–8 hours will be spent on this activity each day. Though perceived physical faults are most frequently found in the skin, hair, or nose, they can impact any body part [9].

Throughout their lives, people with this disorder are typically obsessed with five to seven different body parts. BDD is the idea that one's muscles are too tiny or insufficient. Obsessed with their fantasies, they gaze at the mirror for hours on end, frequently comparing themselves to others. These patients never seem content with their doctor's advice or cosmetic outcomes and often have irrational expectations. A kind of BDD known as BDD via proxy occurs when an individual becomes fixated on the perceived physical shortcomings of other people. It suggests that various factors, including cognitive, psychological, cultural, and biological factors, contribute to the emergence of BDD [10].

Studies have indicated a possible connection between borderline personality disorder and parental emotional, physical, or sexual abuse or neglect. According to one study, those with BDD reported more traumatic early experiences than did healthy controls. Studies show that BDD is three to eight times more common in those with first-degree relatives with these diseases than in the general population, pointing to a potential hereditary component for BDD [11].

BDD affects 0.7% to 2–4% of the overall population. Individuals suffering from additional mental illnesses, such as obsessive-compulsive disorder (OCD), which has a frequency of 8–37%; social phobia patients, 11–13%; substance abuse patients, trichotillomania patients, and anorexia nervosa patients, have higher prevalences of BDD (2–35%). The gender ratio of men to women varies from 1:1 to 3:2 [12].

Among the diagnostic standards are [13]:

1. The person is fixated on one or more imperfections or physical abnormalities that are undetectable to others or only seem minor to them.

2. The person frequently checks himself in the mirror, gives his appearance excessive grooming, or compares it to other people's appearances.

3. The practice seriously impairs one's ability to operate in social, professional, or other domains.

4. The behavior does not fit the criteria for an eating disorder diagnosis.

Typically, BDD symptoms appear in early adolescence. Although the exact cause of BDD is unknown, the majority of its patients have a history of adverse childhood experiences about their body image. Insecurity about one's physique can result from sociocultural factors, such as the exaggerated standards set by performers or models. The four subdivisions of the clinical picture are as follows: 1. issues with appearance; 2. obsessive behavior; 3. functional impairments; 4. a propensity for suicide and self-harm [14].

3. Management of body dysmorphic disorder in cosmetic dermatology

Schut et al. stated that BDD symptoms are more common in patients who come to dermatological practice. It was found that the average participation rate of invited dermatological patients from all 17 countries was 82.4% across all centers. Patients with dermatological issues had five times the prevalence of BDD symptoms (10.5% vs. 2.1%) compared to those with healthy skin controls. Compared to healthy skin controls, patients with dermatological conditions such as vitiligo, hyperhidrosis, and alopecia had an adjusted odds ratio (OR) > 11 times higher chance of experiencing

BDD symptoms. Similarly, patients with psoriasis, acne, Hidradenitis Suppurativa, prurigo, and bullous diseases had an adjusted OR > 6 times higher chance of experiencing BDD symptoms. A logistic regression model revealed a significant relationship between BDD symptoms and female sex, lower age, higher psychological stress, and stigmatization sentiments [15].

Patients with BDD may experience a variety of dermatological problems relating to their skin and hair. Skin pigmentation, acne, scars, excessive body or facial hair, facial asymmetry, thinning scalp hair, and aging symptoms are a few of the issues that surface. They often claim to be highly stressed. They have a history of compulsive behaviors, such as spending hours staring at themselves in the mirror. These patients may also undergo cosmetic surgery, and no matter how nicely the process goes, most of them will never be satisfied with the way they look. It was also shown that women were more likely than men to compare themselves to others when they gazed in the mirror [16].

3.1 Obstacles a dermatologist or cosmetic surgeon may face

Patients with BDD frequently see dermatologists or cosmetologists as their primary point of care. Since many patients are reluctant to talk about the amount of distress they experience as a result of their perceived handicap, it can be difficult to diagnose and recognize BDD. Few people genuinely express their worries and hope that a specific cosmetic operation will significantly improve their lives by fixing obvious flaws. These patients are characterized as having irrational expectations and being "difficult" or "insatiable." These patients also frequently seek the advice of several different physicians, hopping from one to the other until their demands are fulfilled, and their concerns regarding their looks are acknowledged [17].

According to research, some people experience no change at all from medical or surgical procedures intended to improve their appearance, and in certain situations, their problems even get worse. There are multiple accounts of BDD patients harming themselves or filing lawsuits against their physicians for failing to provide acceptable outcomes. The significance of screening patients for BDD or other mental diseases before undergoing medical or surgical intervention is underscored by all of this [18].

The BDD dermatology-questionnaire version (BDDQ-DV), created by Dufresne et al., is a straightforward, adapted method for screening dermatology outpatients. For determining whether BDD is present, this questionnaire has a specificity of 94.7%, sensitivity of 100%, positive predictive value of 70%, and negative predictive value of 100% [19].

The STEP approach, first presented by Elsaie, is another helpful resource for pre-procedure screening. Its use is not restricted to BDD screening, although it helps determine a patient's psychological suitability for cosmetic intervention. "S" stands for stress, and medical professionals use a patient's appearance and behavior to gauge their stress. The letter "T" stands for "target," denoting the area of the body that will be operated on and whether or not the expected outcomes are reasonable. "P" stands for proactive, and "E" stands for envision, or how the patient believes their life will improve following the intervention [20].

Empathy is a vital tool in the counseling of BDD patients. Patients are already under a great deal of stress about their issues. Therefore, brushing them off as unimportant is not a good idea. But it is also not a good idea to concede that they are flawed in any way. Instead, attention should be directed toward understanding their issues, how they impact them, and what kinds of treatments may be provided to help people live better lives. It is also crucial to educate patients on the length of their therapy, the dosage, and any potential adverse effects of the drug they are taking [14].

3.2 Handling

After receiving cosmetic therapy, BDD patients' quality of life (QOL) and self-esteem did not improve, according to research by Wang et al. Because of this, most dermatologists and plastic surgeons decide against treating these individuals in any way. Consequently, most people agree that BDD should be immediately referred for psychiatric management and regarded as a contraindication to cosmetic surgery. As a result, cooperation between these two disciplines is necessary to deliver high-quality treatment [21].

There are not any Food and Drug Administration (FDA) approved drugs for BDD at the moment; the study methodology used to get approval was likely insufficient. Empirical evidence supports first-line methods, including SSRIs, as research-based data is far more limited. Although not recommended by the FDA for BDD, SSRI and CBT are used as the initial treatment strategy in this condition [22].

3.2.1 Serotonin-reuptake inhibitors

Second-generation antidepressants also reduce obsessive thinking and compulsive behavior. Serotonin reuptake inhibitors (SRI) are frequently used to treat a variety of disorders, including major depressive disorder, panic disorder, social anxiety, bulimia, hypochondriasis, post-traumatic stress disorder, and binge eating disorder. SRI can also help with impulsive and anxiety symptoms; on rare occasions, they can even help with pain or violence. The SRI that are currently prescribed in the US are clomipramine (Anafranil), citalopram (Celexa), fluoxetine (Prozac), escitalopram (Lexapro), sertraline (Zoloft), fluvoxamine (Luvox), and paroxetine (Paxil) [22].

Prior studies have demonstrated a substantial increase in compulsive thinking about the objects experienced, a decrease in depressive and anxious symptoms, and an improvement in quality of life among participants in therapy. For BDD, larger dosages of SRI and at least a 12-week course of treatment are typically necessary. Additionally, BDD-related distress and worries about performance faults are lessened with SRI therapy [23].

Studies comparing various SRI dosages for BDD need to be improved; this kind of research is crucial. Our clinical experience suggests that SRI dosages for BDD should be somewhat more significant than those for depression. SRI dosages may be insufficient to treat BDD, if medical professionals solely address depression symptoms adequately. Phillips employed escitalopram 29 ± 12 mg/day, citalopram 66 ± 36 mg/day, fluoxetine 67 ± 24 mg/day, and fluoxetine 308 ± 49 mg/day as average doses in the clinical practice [22]. Some people may benefit from using SRI higher than the maximum dosages advised by the pharmaceutical firm, such as escitalopram 50 mg/day, citalopram 80–100 mg/day, fluvoxamine 400 mg/day, or fluvoxamine 300 mg/day. However, the dose of Clomipramine should not exceed 250 mg per day. Various factors will determine the speed of increasing the dose. For patients who are genuinely ill or suicidal, it is best to titrate more quickly; however, titration also depends on patient preference, how well the medication is tolerated, and how often they contact their doctor. It is difficult to judge whether lower doses are beneficial. However, slower titrations may have the disadvantage of being unnecessary and protracted. Based on the patient's condition, SRI titration modifications must be made [24].

Typically, the effects of SRI take time to manifest and may take anywhere from 12 to 16 weeks. So, treatment should be carried out for more than 16 weeks. SRI therapy is effective if it is continued for several years or even longer. There are not any significant risks to continuing SRI for many years. Patients who experience relapse after SRI discontinuation are good candidates for long-term SRI treatment [22].

Patients who stop receiving effective SRI medication will relapse over the next 6 months; therefore, caution is required while ending SRI therapy [24]. In patients who frequently relapse, their function and QoL are significantly impaired [25]. Treatment discontinuation can occur for several reasons, such as side effects, lack of access to treatment, or the desire to be free from medication. SRI should, however, be decreased gradually over a few months rather than all at once. Do not think that if you get CBT while on an SRI, it will lessen your chance of relapsing after you quit the medication. Redistributing SRI did not elicit the same strong reaction as the initial trial [22].

The adverse effects may be connected to the dose size administered because the SRI used in BDD may be more than in other diseases. SRI side effects are frequently manageable and often go away with time. When first prescribed, patients should be made aware of this. It is necessary to modify the dosage if adverse effects arise. Sedation or activation, sleeplessness, gastrointestinal symptoms including nausea and delayed orgasm, and symptoms like vivid dreams or dizziness after stopping an SRI are some of the side effects that are linked to these medications. Therefore, titrating slowly up or down when adjusting the dose is a good idea [26].

3.2.2 Cognitive behavioral therapy

According to the cognitive-behavioral model for borderline personality disorder, individuals with BDD exhibit repetitive activities as coping methods, such as checking mirrors and avoiding social situations, and focus their entire sense of self-worth on insignificant appearance defects. CBT aims to help the patient overcome their problematic thought patterns and behaviors by using cognitive restructuring and psychoeducation. One to five CBT sessions per week, lasting one to one-and-a-half hours, are administered for several weeks. It can be given as group CBT or one-on-one [27].

Assessment of BDD and associated symptoms is the first step in CBT. Physicians ought to inquire about BDD-related diseases, thoughts, actions, and body parts of concern. Asking about BDD symptoms is crucial because shyness frequently prevents them from being recognized in clinical settings [28]. Clinical practitioners should be on the lookout for clues in the patient's appearance (e.g., skin peeling scars) and behavior (e.g., wearing camouflage) to conceal the condition; what the patient finds disturbing (e.g., feelings when people talk about them, stare at them); panic attacks (e.g., when looking in the mirror); depression; social anxiety; drug abuse; suicidal thoughts; and inability to remain at home. Furthermore, in a systematic clinical interview, differential diagnoses such as depression, social anxiety, eating disorders, and obsessive-compulsive disorder should be clarified. It is essential to screen for depression and suicidality early in treatment and regularly due to the high incidence of both conditions in BDD patients.

Therapists should utilize motivational interviewing [29] approaches that have been adapted for use in borderline personality disorder with patients who are unwilling to undergo CBT or whose ideas seem excessively delusional. Instead of immediately challenging the patient's views, the therapist should first show empathy for the patient's misery connected to body image ("I see that you are suffering because you are very worried about your appearance"). Let us attempt to lessen this anxiety. Furthermore, non-judgmental Socratic inquiries such as "What are the benefits of trying CBT for BDD?" might be employed as delusional [30].

The therapist should then provide psychoeducation about BDD, including its frequency, typical symptoms, and the differences between body image and appearance. After that, based on the latter's particular symptoms, the patient and the therapist develop a personalized BDD model. Theories concerning the biological, social, and psychological elements that lead to the development of body image problems are included in these models. It is critical to assess patients' circumstances to determine what sustains their issues with body image. These elements include emotional reactions, triggers for unfavorable appearance-related beliefs, interpreting these thoughts, and (maladaptive) coping mechanisms. This will help determine the essential modules and the course of treatment. Cognitive strategies include recognizing, evaluating, and generating alternative beliefs. The therapist exposes the patient to common mental errors associated with BDD, like "mind reading" and "all-or-nothing thinking." Following that, patients are urged to keep an eye on their thought processes based on how they seem inside and outside sessions and recognize cognitive errors [30].

Therapists can begin assessing the patient's thoughts once they can recognize their cognitive errors and maladaptive thoughts. False core beliefs must be addressed after the patient recognizes and reframes instinctive ideas about their appearance. "I am incapable" or "I am unlovable" are typical core beliefs in BDD. In therapy, core beliefs often emerge. Cognitive restructuring, behavioral experiments, and self-esteem-building techniques effectively overcome negative underlying beliefs. These techniques teach patients to broaden the scope of their self-esteem beyond appearance values, such as ability, achievement, and morality [31].

The therapist and patient should review the patient's BDD model before starting Preventing exposure and rituals (PE/R) to help identify the patient's rituals (such as excessive mirror checking), avoidance behaviors (such as avoiding traveling the subway), and the purpose behind those rituals. Together, the patient and therapist create a hierarchy of anxiety-inducing and -avoidance circumstances. Patients frequently shy away from everyday tasks that can highlight their alleged shortcomings. Scenarios that will broaden the patient's social experience in general should be included in the hierarchy. The therapist can advise going out twice a week with friends rather than shunning them on days when she thinks her nose is particularly "big" [32].

The patient typically concentrates solely on the area of his body that bothers him and is too near the mirror, exaggerating perceived flaws and perpetuating maladaptive BDD behaviors. Patients who undergo perceptual retraining are able to overcome incorrect impressions of their bodies and acquire healthy mirror-related behaviors (e.g., refraining from approaching mirrors too closely or avoiding them entirely). When the patient is standing a conversational distance away from the mirror—two to three feet, for example—the therapist assists them in describing their entire body, from head to toe. During perceptual (mirror) retraining, patients learn to describe themselves more objectively, such as "There is a small bump on the bridge of my nose," as opposed to using judgmental language, such as "My nose is big and crooked."

Therapists advise their clients not to engage in ritualistic behaviors like caressing or dozing off in uncomfortable spots. Patients are urged to work on focusing on other aspects of their surroundings, such as the flavor of the food and the conversations that they hear, rather than how they look or how other people seem [30].

Psychoeducation and cognitive behavioral techniques specifically designed to address shape/weight concerns are often beneficial for patients with considerable concerns about their appearance, including those with muscle dysmorphia. Therapists can assist patients in weighing the advantages and disadvantages of cosmetic surgery without passing judgment by using cognitive and motivational techniques to dispel maladaptive ideas about the benefits of surgery. Patients with BDD frequently experience depression, which might complicate their care [30].

3.2.3 Electroconvulsive therapy

Electroconvulsive therapy, or ECT, involves applying electricity to the brain. The main conditions that ECT is used to treat include schizophrenia, bipolar disorder, and major depressive disorder (MDD). ECT is not mentioned as a substitute treatment for OCD that is recalcitrant, albeit [33]. In reality, ECT-related deaths are a very rare event [34]. The primary reason is a deficiency of evidence-based data [35]. In recent years, ECT has drawn more interest as a treatment for OCD. In a prior trial, it was only judged to be helpful in two out of 25 instances and was limited to individuals with severe depression who were contemplating suicide. Surgical methods such as modified leukotomy, capsulotomy, subcaudate tractotomy, and bilateral anterior cingulotomy are the last resort when no other treatments work to relieve severe symptoms of BDD [23]. In individuals with BDD comorbidity, ECT may be safely used to treat a major depressive episode that is resistant to treatment. ECT potentially improves both depressive and body dysmorphic symptoms [36].

4. Conclusion

One way to think of somatization is as a process that essentially develops as a coping mechanism for stress. Somatosensory amplification is another idea where somatic sensations are perceived as severe, frightening, or unsettling. There are three components to somatization. (i) Hypervigilance (to bodily sensations); (ii) specificity (to weak sensations); and (iii) intensification (to make them more concerning) through affect and cognition. Recurrent subjective feelings of physical symptoms (henceforth referred to as somatoform symptoms) that are unrelated to any physical illness are the hallmark of somatoform diseases. One characteristic unites all these illnesses' subtypes: the preponderance and persistence of somatic symptoms linked to significant suffering and impairment.

Most BDD patients first see a cosmetic outpatient because the disorder is underdiagnosed and misdiagnosed. When their demands are not met, they may feel unsatisfied with their cosmetic procedures and may resort to violence or take legal action against the practitioner. This illness highlights how crucial it is for dermatologists and cosmetic surgeons to understand BDD and be prepared with screening techniques to recognize cases as soon as possible and refer patients to a colleague who works in psychology. Consequently, to treat BDD patients holistically, the two specialists need to collaborate.

Acknowledgements

We would like to express our gratitude to Farida Ulfa for her timely and efficient collaboration. Her dedication, professionalism, and prompt response to queries have made the research process smoother and more efficient.

Conflict of interest

The authors declare no conflict of interest.

Appendices and nomenclature

BDD	body dysmorphic disorder
BDDQ-DV	BDD dermatology-questionnaire version
BSI	Bradford somatic inventory
CBT	cognitive behavioral therapy
DSM V	diagnostic and statistical manual of mental disorders, fifth edition
FDA	Food and Drug Administration
IAD	illness anxiety disorder
IAS	illness attitude scale
ICD-10	International Classification of Diseases, 10th Edition
MBCT	mindfulness-based cognitive therapy
PHQ-15	Patient Health Questionnaire-15
QoL	quality of life
SASS-R	the scale for assessment of somatic symptoms
SNRIs	serotonin and norepinephrine reuptake inhibitors
SRI	serotonin reuptake inhibitor
SSRI	selective serotonin reuptake inhibitor
SSD	somatic symptom disorder
SSS	somatic symptom scale
SSS-8	Somatic Symptom Scale-8
WI	The Whiteley Index

Author details

Dian Andriani Ratna Dewi[1,2]*, Amin Ibrizatun[1], Lila Irawati Tjahjo Widuri[1], Hayra Avianggi[2] and Fakhira Ayu Wijayanti[1]

1 The Republic of Indonesia Defense University, Bogor, Indonesia

2 Army Central Hospital Gatot Soebroto, Jakarta, Indonesia

*Address all correspondence to: dianandrianiratnadewi@gmail.com

References

[1] Witthöft M, Jasper F, Hennemann S. Somatic symptom disorder. In: Encyclopedia of Mental Health. 3rd ed. Academic Press; 2023. pp. V3-336-V3-342. DOI: 10.1016/B978-0-323-91497-0.00118-1

[2] Agarwal V, Srivastava C. Clinical practice guidelines for the management of somatoform disorders in children and adolescents. Indian Journal of Psychiatry. 2019;**2019**(Suppl. 2):62-71. DOI: 10.4103/psychiatry.IndianJPsychiatry_775_19

[3] Alanazi AO, Aljohani RA, Aljohani MF, Alhussaini AA, Alnemer FK, et al. Epidemiological features and clinical manifestations of patients with somatoform disorder at a tertiary Medical City in Riyadh, Saudi Arabia. Cureus. 2021;**13**(11):11-19. DOI: 10.7759/cureus.19799

[4] Agarwal V, Nischal A, Praharaj SK, Menon V. Clinical practice guideline: Psychotherapies for somatoform disorders. Indian Journal of Psychiatry. 2020;**62**(Suppl):263-227. DOI: 10.4103/psychiatry.IndianJPsychiatry_775_19

[5] Pavithra N, Dahale AB, Desai G. Hypochondriasis: Clinical profile in a tertiary care psychiatry and neurosciences hospital in Southern India – A retrospective chart review. Indian Journal of Psychological Medicine. 2019;**41**(2):178-181. DOI: 10.4103/IJPSYM.IJPSYM_177_18

[6] Chappell AS. Toward a lifestyle medicine approach to illness anxiety disorder (formerly hypochondriasis). American Journal of Lifestyle Medicine. 2018;**12**(5):365-369. DOI: 10.1177/1559827618764649

[7] Newby JM, Hobbs MJ, Mahoney AEJ, Wong S(K), Andrews G. DSM-5 illness anxiety disorder and somatic symptom disorder: Comorbidity, correlates, and overlap with DSM-IV hypochondriasis. Journal of Psychosomatic Research. 2017;**101**:31-37. DOI: 10.1016/j.jpsychores.2017.07.010

[8] Sansone RA, Sansone LA. Serotonin norepinephrine reuptake inhibitors: A pharmacological comparison. Innovations in Clinical Neuroscience. 2014;**11**(3-4):37-42

[9] Phillips KA, Dufresne RG. Body dysmorphic disorder a guide for dermatologists and cosmetic surgeons. American Journal of Clinical Dermatology. 2000;**1**(4):235-243. DOI: 10.2165/00128071-200001040-00005

[10] Singh AR, Veale D. Understanding and treating body dysmorphic disorder. Indian Journal of Psychiatry. 2019;**2019**:131-135. DOI: 10.4103/psychiatry.indianJPsychiatry_528_18

[11] Feusner JD, Neziroglu F, Wilhelm S, Mancusi L, Bohon C. What causes BDD: Research findings and a proposed model. Psychiatric Annals. 2010;**40**(7):349-355. DOI: 10.3928/00485713-20100701-08

[12] Phillips KA, Menard W, Fay C. Gender similarities and differences in 200 individuals with body dysmorphic disorder. Comprehensive Psychiatry. 2006;**47**(2):77-87. DOI: 10.1016/j.comppsych.2005.07.002

[13] Schieber K, Kollei K, De Zwaan M, Martin A. Classification of body dysmorphic disorder — What is the advantage of the new DSM-5 criteria ? Journal of Psychosomatic Research. 2015;**78**(3):223-227. DOI: 10.1016/j.jpsychores.201 5.01.002

[14] Shivakumar S, Jafferany M, Sood S, Susruth V. Cosmetic presentations and challenges of body dysmorphic disorder and its collaborative management. Journal of Cutaneous and Aesthetic Surgery. 2021;**14**(1):20-25. DOI: 10.4103/JCAS.JCAS_180_20

[15] Schut C, Dalgard FJ, Bewley A, Evers AWM, Gieler U, et al. Body dysmorphia in common skin disease: Results of an observational, cross sectional multicentre study among dermatological outpatients in 17 European countries. British Journal of Dermatology. 2022;**187**:115-125. DOI: 10.1111/BJD.21021

[16] Koran LM, Hanna GL, Hollander E, Nestadt G, Simpson HB, American Psychiatric Association. Practice guideline for the treatment of patients with obsessive-compulsive disorder. American Journal of Psychiatry. 2007;**164**(7 Suppl):5-53

[17] Sarwer DB. Awareness and identification of body dysmorphic disorder by aesthetic surgeons: Results of a survey of American Society for Aesthetic Plastic Surgery Members. Aesthetic Surgery Journal. 2002;**22**(6):531-535. DOI: 10.1067/maj.2002.129451

[18] Sweis IE, Spitz J, Barry DR Jr, Cohen M. A review of body dysmorphic disorder in aesthetic surgery patients and the legal implications. Aesthetic Plastic Surgery. 2017;**41**(4):949-954. DOI: 10.1007/s00266-017-0819-x

[19] Dufresne RG, Phillips KA, Vittorio CC, Wilkel CS. A screening questionnaire for body dysmorphic disorder in a cosmetic dermatologic surgery practice. Dermatologic Surgery. 2001;**27**(5):457-462. DOI: 10.1046/J.1524-4725.2002.00190.x

[20] Elsaie ML. Psychological approach in cosmetic dermatology for optimum patient satisfaction. Indian Journal of Dermatology. 2010;(55):127-129. DOI: 10.4103/0019-5154.62733

[21] Wang Q, Cao C, Guo R, Li X, Lu L, et al. Avoiding psychological pitfalls in aesthetic medical procedures. Aesthetic Plastic Surgery. 2016;**40**(6):954-961. DOI: 10.1007/s00266-016-0715-9

[22] Phillips KA, Hollander E. Treating body dysmorphic disorder with medication: Evidence, misconceptions, and a suggested approach. Body Image. 2008;**5**(1):13-27. DOI: 10.1016/j.bodyim.2007.12.003

[23] Phillips KA. Pharmacotherapy for body dysmorphic disorder. Psychiatric Annals. 2016;**40**(7):325-332. DOI: 10.3928/00485713-20100701-05

[24] Phillips KA, Menard W, Fay C. Demographiccharateristics,phenomenology, comorbidity and family history in 200 individuals with body dysmorphic disorder. Psycosomatics. 2005;**15**(10):1203-1214. DOI: 10.1176/appi.psy.46.4.317

[25] Hollander E, Stein DJ, Fineberg NA, Marteau F, Legault. Quality of life outcomes in patients with obsessive-compulsive disorder. The Journal of Clinical Psychiatry. 2010;**71**(06):784-792. DOI: 10.4088/jcp.09m05911blu

[26] Rabiei Z, Rabie Z. A review on antidepressant effect of medicinal plants. Bangladesh Journal of Pharmacology. 2017;**12**(1):1-11. DOI: 10.3329/bjp.v12i1.29184

[27] Prazeres AM, Nascimento AL, Fontenelle LF. Cognitive-behavioral therapy for body dysmorphic disorder: A review of its efficacy. Neuropsychiatric Disease and Treatment. 2013;**9**:307-316. DOI: 10.2147/NDT.S41074

[28] Conroy M, Menard W, Fleming-Ives K, Modha P, Cerullo H, Phillips KA. Prevalence and clinical characteristics of body dysmorphic disorder in an adult inpatient setting. General Hospital Psychiatry. 2008;**30**(1):67-72. DOI: 10.1016/j.genhosppsych.2007.09.004

[29] Randall CL, McNeil DW. Motivational interviewing as an adjunct to cognitive behavior therapy for anxiety disorders: A critical review of the literature. Cognitive and Behavioral Practice. 2017;**24**(3):296-311. DOI: 10.1016/j.cbpra.2016.05.003

[30] Wilhelm S, Phillips KA, Didie E, Buhlmann U, Greenberg JL, et al. Modular cognitive-behavioral therapy for body dysmorphic disorder: A randomized controlled trial. Behavior Therapy. 2014;**45**(3):314-327. DOI: 10.1016/j.beth.2013.12.007

[31] Veale D. Advances in a cognitive behavioural model of body dysmorphic disorder. Body Image. 2004;**1**(1):113-125. DOI: 10.1016/S1740-1445(03)00009-3

[32] Gunstad J, Phillips KA. Axis I comorbidity in body dysmorphic disorder. Comprehensive Psychiatry. 2006;**44**(4):270-276. DOI: 10.1016/S0010-440X(03)00088-9

[33] Kellner CH, Obbels J, Sienaert P. When to consider electroconvulsive therapy (ECT). Acta Psychiatrica Scandinavica. 2020;**141**(4):304-315. DOI: 10.1111/acps.13134

[34] Tørring N, Sanghani SN, Petrides G, Kellner CH, Østergaard SD. The mortality rate of electroconvulsive therapy: A systematic review and pooled analysis. Acta Psychiatrica Scandinavica. 2017;**135**(5):388-397. DOI: 10.1111/acps.12721

[35] Xiang YT, Ungar GS, Correll CU, Chiu HFK, Lai KYC, et al. Use of electroconvulsive therapy for Asian patients with schizophrenia (2001-2009): Trends and correlates. Psychiatry and Clinical Neurosciences. 2015;**69**(8):489-496. DOI: 10.1111/pcn.12283

[36] Rapinesi C, Serata D, Del Casale A, Carbonetti P, Fensore C, et al. Effectiveness of electroconvulsive therapy in a patient with a treatment-resistant major depressive episode and comorbid body dysmorphic disorder. The Journal of ECT. 2013;**29**(2):145-146. DOI: 10.1097/YCT.0b013e31827ce88e